Spiralizer 101

Gluten-Free
VEGETABLE
Spiralizer
COOKBOOK

*101 GLUTEN-FREE RECIPES THAT TURN
VEGETABLES INTO DELICIOUSLY SATISFYING
MEALS USING PADERNO, VEGGETTI, IPERFECT, &
BRIEFTONS SPIRALIZERS.*

Tom Anderson

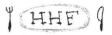

HHF Press
San Francisco

1

LEGAL NOTICE

The information contained in this book is for entertainment purposes only. The content represents the opinion of the author and is based on the author's personal experience and observations. The author does not assume any liability whatsoever for the use of or inability to use any or all information contained in this book, and accepts no responsibility for any loss or damages of any kind that may be incurred by the reader as a result of actions arising from the use of information in this book. Use this information at your own risk.

The author reserves the right to make any changes he or she deems necessary to future versions of the publication to ensure its accuracy.

PRAISE FROM READERS...

"This is a great book for vegetable spiralizer owners, and people who are interested in substituting vegetable "pasta" in place of traditional wheat pasta. The author, J.S. Amie, seems to have a good following on Amazon, and after reading this book I can see why!"

- Michelle G.

"My son has Celiac disease so we have to get creative in avoiding gluten. The Spiralizer really helps but the problem is, I'm just not that creative in the kitchen! My son isn't crazy about straight up string zucchini which is where this book comes in. It offers inventive and creative recipes that I never would have come up with and my son (who is 11) will actually eat without complaint. He still seems to complains about everything else."

- Ryan J.

"Really happy with this book. Not only do you get delicious recipes, but you also can instruction on how to properly use your Paderno. I am trying to limit my gluten and wheat intake and my diet is mostly Paleo at this point, so these recipes are perfect!"

- Mary T.

"Its a very handy book to have. It gives suggestions on what kind of vegetables and fruits to use and how to clean your spiralizer.

- Renee I.

"This is a great intro into spiralizers. It has some great healthy gluten free, paleo and weight loss recipes. The Chicken Curry with Cauliflower "Rice" is on the menu tonight!"

- Dip F.

"Great book with quick and easy recipes. I was disappointed that the Paderno itself didn't come with any type of book, but I'm glad I ordered this."

- Hammer

GET THE QUICKSTART GUIDE FREE!

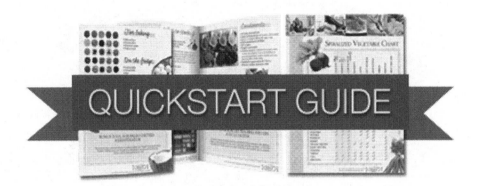

This book comes with a Spiralized Vegetable Quickstart Guide which includes:

- Which Vegetables To Use
- Pro Spiralizing Techniques
- Gluten-free, Paleo, and Weight-Loss Pantry Charts
- Free recipe resources

We've found that readers have more success with our book when they use the Quickstart Guide. Download it today...absolutely free! See Chapter 9 for details.

DO YOU LIKE FREE BOOKS?

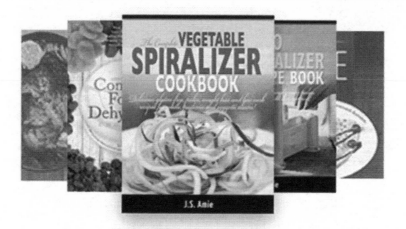

Every month we release a new book, and we offer it to our current readers first...absolutely free! This helps us get early feedback before launching a book, and lets you stock your shelf full of interesting and valuable books for free!

Some recent titles include:

- The Weight Loss Vegetable Spiralizer Cookbook
- The French Crepe Cookbook
- The Food Dehydrator Handbook

To receive this month's free book, just go to

www.healthyhappyfoodie.org/b1-freebooks

TABLE OF CONTENTS

CHAPTER 1: WHY YOU NEED THIS COOKBOOK 11

CHAPTER 2: WHAT IS "SPIRALIZING"? 13

CHAPTER 3: 7 REASONS TO SPIRALIZE FOR LIFE 15

CHAPTER 4: THE BEST SPIRALIZERS 19

CHAPTER 5: HOW TO MAKE SPIRALIZED NOODLES & RICE 33

CHAPTER 6: HOW TO CHOOSE THE BEST VEGETABLES
(AND FRUITS) FOR SPIRALIZING 39

CHAPTER 7: 8 WAYS TO COOK THE PERFECT SPIRALIZED DISH 43

CHAPTER 8: SPIRALIZING TIPS 49

CHAPTER 9: HOW TO USE THIS BOOK 51

CHAPTER 10: SOUPS 53

    Asian Pasta with Broth 54
    Black Bean & Noodle Soup 56
    Butternut Squash Avocado Soup 58
    Curried Leek & Lentil Soup 60
    Green Chile, Chicken, Squash Soup 62
    Mexican Chicken Noodle Soup 64
    Mexican Tomato Soup with Squash Noodles 66
    Gluten Free Miso Noodle Soup 68
    Pork & Noodle Soup with Greens 70
    Pumpkin Noodle Soup 72
    Rosemary Root Vegetable Soup 74
    Shoyu Cabbage Soup 76
    Shrimp Soup with Bok Choy 78
    Sizzling "Rice" Soup 80
    Slow - Cooker Minestrone 82
    Thai Chicken Noodle Soup 84

Tunisian Noodle Soup 86

CHAPTER 11: SALADS 87

Asian Chicken & Noodle Salad 88
Beet Salad 90
Beef Salad 91
Light Citrus Ginger Tofu Salad with Carrot and Squash Noodles 92
Colorful Carrot & Beet Slaw 95
Greek Pasta Salad 96
Mediterranean Pasta Salad 98
Noodles & Humus Salad 100
One Pot Kale and Cauliflower Pilaf 102
Pasta Primavera Salad 104
Roasted Baby Turnips with Dijon-Shallot Vinaigrette and Beet Noodles
.... 106
Shaved Asparagus, Yellow Squash, and Mint Salad 108
Vegetables with Rosemary Vinaigrette 110
Zucchini and Squash Summer Salad with Golden Raisins, Pistachios, and Mint 112
Zucchini, Squash, and Spinach Salad with Apples and Cranberries 114
South of the Border Jicama-Avocado Salad 116
Dill Salmon Pasta Salad 117
Thai Green Papaya Salad 118

CHAPTER 12: SIDES 119

Potato-Veggie Latkes 120
Baked Zucchini and Potato Pancakes 122
Cabbage and Apple Sauté 124
Curried Vegetable Couscous 126
French Peasant Beets Spirals 128
Lemon Chard Pasta 130
Mediterranean Squash Stir-fry 132
Mexican Slaw 134
Perfumed Noodles with Fruit & Nuts 136
Southwestern Spiced Sweet Potato and Beet Spirals with Chilli-Cilantro Sour Cream 138
Spicy Slaw 140
Sesame Noodles 141
Squash Sauté 142

Roasted Vegetable Snacks 144

CHAPTER 13: MAIN DISHES 145

Baked Chicken Parmesan with Noodles 146
Baked Eggs with Spiralized Jicama 148
Beef Paprikash with Squash Noodles 150
Beef Pho 152
Cabbage and Apple Sauté 154
Cabbage "Spaghetti" with Turkey Sauce 156
Chicken Curry with Cauliflower "Rice" 158
Chicken Veggie Alfredo 160
Chili Cincinnati Style 162
Curried Chicken with Pasta 164
Drunken Clams with Sausage 166
"Drunken Noodles" with Chicken 168
Ethiopian-Inspired Spicy Chicken Stew 170
Florentine Potato Pasta Casserole 172
Funky Low Fat Chicken With Sesame Noodles 174
Greek Lamb Pasta 176
Pasta & Turkey/Chia Seed Meatballs 178
Pasta Cajun Style 180
Pasta e Fagilo 182
Pasta Puttanesca 184
Pasta with Anchovy Sauce 186
Pasta with Charred Tomato Sauce 188
Pasta with Clams 190
Pesto Zucchini Pasta with Sausage 192
Pizza Pasta 194
Porcini and Rosemary Crusted Beef Tenderloin with Port Wine Sauce
and Potato Linguini 196
Quick and Easy Pasta Arrabiata 200
Quick and Easy Pasta with Lemon & Ricott 202
Rosemary Pork Ragout with Sweet Potato Pasta 204
Secret Ingredient Beef Stew 206
Slow Cooker Zucchini Pasta With Eggplant Sauce 208
Smoked Salmon Pasta with Lemon & Dill 210
Spicy Shrimp with Vegetable Noodles and Baby Spinach 212
Spicy Vegetable Noodles with Kale and Peanut Sauce 214
Squash and Zucchini Pasta with Prosciutto, Snap Peas, and Mint 216

Squash Noodles with Tomatoes and Turkey Bacon.................................218
Squash Sauté...220
Sweet Potato Pasta with Asparagus and Pancetta 222
Tomato-Bacon Squash Pasta..224
Red Wine-Braised Short Ribs with Roasted Turnips 226
Turkey Pho...229
Turkey Pie with Spaghetti Crust...232
Turkey Ragu and Potato Pasta Bake..234
Vegetable Mock-Fried "Rice" 236
Zucchini Pasta Ala Checca..238
Greek Lamb with Riced Cauliflower 240

CHAPTER 14: DESSERTS...**243**

Apple Crisp 244
Apple Ribbon Pie with Nut Crust...246
Apple/Rhubarb Compote 248
Fried Apples 250
Sweet Potato Pudding..251

CHAPTER 15: NEXT STEPS...**253**

ABOUT THE AUTHOR **254**

1

WHY YOU NEED THIS COOKBOOK

LEARN HOW TO USE YOUR SPIRALIZER LIKE A PRO

What do your local greasy spoon and your favorite restaurant have in common? They both work with the same basic ingredients. What makes your favorite restaurant's meals so much more appetizing (and probably pricier)? Know-how and recipes. In this book you'll learn how to use your new spiralizer like a pro, and how to make the most delicious spiralizer recipes imaginable. Ready to start?

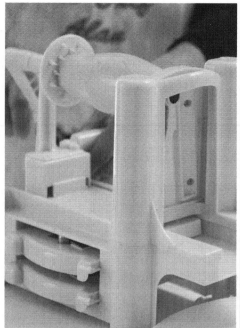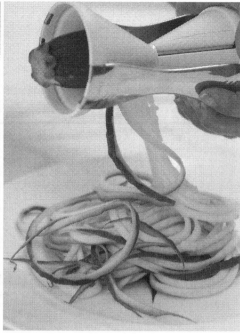

HELP ACHIEVING YOUR GLUTEN-FREE LIFESTYLE GOALS

Which forbidden food do you crave most? If you're like many adhering to a gluten-free lifestyle, "pasta" is the answer. That's why this book contains so many recipes mimicking traditional Italian and American pasta dishes.

A BLUEPRINT FOR A HEALTHY LIFESTYLE

Spiralizing allows you to "have your pasta and eat it too." You can now enjoy many of the pasta dishes you grew up with and love, but in a way that supports your healthy lifestyle. This book was written with you in mind. Give it a try, you'll love it ☺

2

WHAT IS "SPIRALIZING"?

"Spiralizing" is a new cooking trend that has revolutionized the way many people prepare their meals. Spiralizing is literally the process of slicing fresh vegetables and fruits into spiral-shaped strands which have a size and texture similar to pasta. While the concept is simple, the result is surprisingly rich, flavorful, and versatile.

Once you become skilled with a spiralizer, you can replace wheat pasta in almost any existing pasta dish with fresh zucchini noodles (or carrot noodles, sweet potato, squash, etc). You will feel liberated from heavy, high-carb meals. You will have joined the revolution.

Like so many life-changing movements, the "spiralizing revolution" began with a simple idea—a clever kitchen gadget that would allow cooks to make quick and delicious substitutes for fattening dishes that were ruining their health and appearance.

Because spiralizing was not just fun but easy, using the spiral-cut vegetables quickly became a hot, foodie trend. The "spiralizer" movement gained momentum as influencers in different dietary communities—carnivores, omnivores, vegetarians, raw foodists, you name it—began praising the healthful benefits of adding spiral-cut vegetables to their menus.

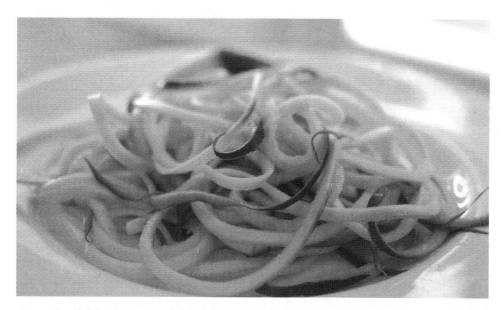

Soon food bloggers and cookbook authors were singing the praises of the spiralizers and the benefits of using spiral-cut vegetables in every kind of cuisine. Spiralized vegetables showed up on the plates of trendy restaurants and in the dining rooms of trend-setting home cooks interested in a new way to eat healthier. And the trend continued to spread as the benefits of this new, clean, green way of eating became obvious—better health, weight-loss, and an overall increase in well-being.

3

7 REASONS TO SPIRALIZE FOR LIFE

Besides being naturally gluten-free, spiralized vegetables offer many health and emotional benefits:

SPIRALIZING LEADS TO BETTER HEALTH

Nutritionists have long made a connection between "inflammatory" foods and illness ranging from "leaky gut syndrome" to cancer. Simple carbs are high on the "inflammatory" scale and eating too many carbs too often keeps the body in a constant state of "irritation" that eventually results in illness. One small dietary change like substituting vegetable strands for pasta will pay off in big health rewards.

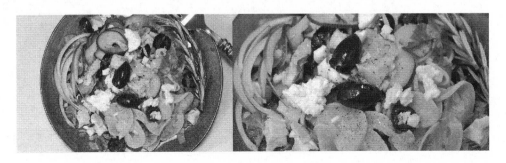

EASY WAY TO REPLACE WHEAT IN EVERYDAY MEALS

Craving a big plate of comforting, old-fashioned, gluten-saturated pasta? Now you can satisfy that craving easily and quickly by replacing pasta with fresh, nutritious, gluten-free spiralized vegetables! Spiralizing is the easiest and quickest way to enjoy the delicious traditional flavors and textures of Italian pasta without paying the price of gluten reaction. Now, anytime you want traditional pasta, just pull out your spiralizer and enjoy!

SPIRALIZING MAKES IT EASIER TO LOSE WEIGHT

Pasta, potatoes, and processed foods make up the bad nutrition trifecta. Whether consumed as a "comfort food" (French fries, macaroni and cheese) or as a high-calorie, high-carb meal like a traditional Italian feast with pasta and garlic bread, low-quality carbs cause blood-sugar spikes that stress out the body's endocrine system, resulting in hormonal ups and downs that lead to everything from added body fat to an increased potential for developing Type II diabetes, heart, disease, and other deadly conditions.

EASY WAY TO ADD MORE NUTRITION

The standard American diet is filled with empty calories and junk food. The complex interconnection of blood-sugar and satiety levels can lead to "chain-eating' and over-indulging because the body's natural triggers that signal "fullness" have been disabled.

With spiralized vegetable strands, the body can process a meal the way food was meant to be processed, using it for fuel without storing it as fat, and allowing the nourishment of vegetables to replenish the body's tissues rather than plumping them out with extra glucose caused by a massive overload of pasta.

FAMILY-FRIENDLY LOW-CARB MEALS

Children love the colorful vegetable strands created by spiralizers, so adding them to your daily meals is a painless, delicious way to get your kids to "eat their greens." With childhood obesity at an all-time high, that's an important goal to achieve. Not only that, but the recipes in this book will introduce you to a variety of dishes that will add pizazz to mealtimes without adding empty calories.

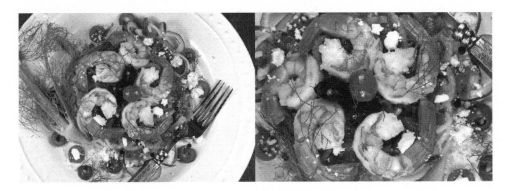

WORKS WITH ANY DIET

Spiralized vegetables and fruits fit into any dietary plan—from raw foo diets to eating plans as disparate as veganism and Paleo. With spiralized vegetables, the household cook won't be making different meals in order to accommodate different family members.

ADD NEW TEXTURES & FLAVORS TO YOUR MEALS

Spiralized vegetables and fruits offer a large variety of new flavors and textures to a tired-out repertoire. From soft, tender zucchini strands to crispy cauliflower rice...Once you try, you'll never go back!

4

THE BEST SPIRALIZERS

Using the right tool for the job is—as any handyman/woman knows—the key to success; you don't use a hammer to tighten a screw. There are three kinds of vegetable slicers on the market, and all have strengths and weaknesses you should be aware of when making a choice. (Or buy all three and have options!)

VEGGETTI – STYLE SPIRALIZERS

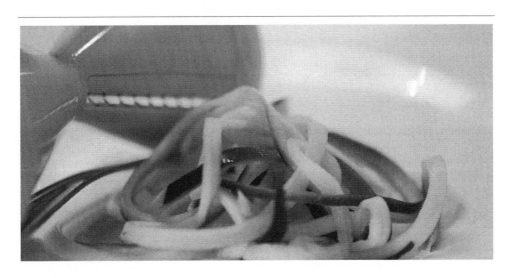

Best for: quick set up, small quantities of noodles, small "footprint" on the counter, and traveling.

This inventive, hourglass-shaped kitchen utensil is easy to use, easy to clean, and lightweight enough to carry with you when you travel. If you can imagine a pencil sharpener large enough to accommodate a zucchini, then you've just imagined the Veggetti Spiral Vegetable Slicer and how it works.

As with anything in your kitchen that has a blade—blender, food processor, silverware drawer— the Veggetti can bite if you're not careful. The blades are extremely sharp, so you need to be alert while you're turning your vegetables into delicious, low-calorie spaghetti strands. Most mishaps occur when a hand slips while guiding the vegetable through the blades, or when someone sticks a finger into the blade during cleaning.

Keep in mind that very little force is necessary. All you need to do is gently twist your vegetables through, preferably using the Veggetti's cap to grip the vegetable while you're twisting it.

Here's How To Use The Veggetti Safely:

STEP 1: Leave the skin on the gripping end of the vegetable. This gives you a more solid and less slippery surface to grip while you're twisting the vegetable into the Veggetti.

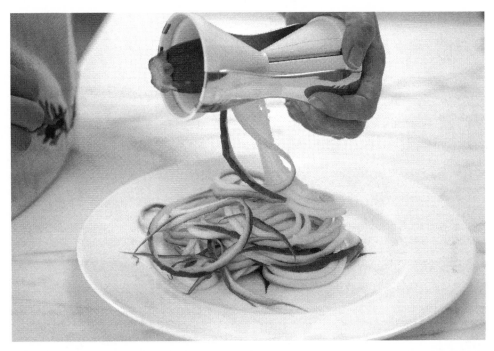

Notes: For most vegetables—such as zucchinis, carrots, yellow squash—I simply grip the end of the vegetable with my hand. However, the Veggetti comes with a "cap" that has little spikes which help to grip slippery vegetables. I find that this cap works well for dense vegetables (carrots), but not for soft vegetables (zucchini). In my experience, the cap will shred the end of soft vegetables, making it even more difficult to push them through the Veggetti. Another option to get the last inch of goodness out of each vegetable, is to stab a fork into the vegetable instead of using your fingers or the cap.

STEP 2: the Veggetti cutter looks like an hourglass with two open ends. Each "funnel" has a different blade so that you can vary the type of vegetable pasta you get—spaghetti-type strands or wider, udon noodles. Choose the width of noodle you want and guide your vegetable into that blade.

Notes: You'll quickly develop a preference for either the spaghetti or the udon noodle size for each vegetable. I love both, depending on the dish. Generally, I prefer the thinner spaghetti noodles for denser vegetables (carrots, beets, etc). For raw or lightly cooked dishes, I also prefer the thinner spaghetti noodles. However, the thicker udon noodles are great for soups, or dishes with thick sauces.

STEP 3: Once your vegetable is cleaned, scrubbed, or peeled, simply place the end you want to cut into the Veggetti and begin turning it, just as you would when sharpening a pencil. The "pasta" strands will begin appearing as soon as the turning starts. Discard the left over portion of the vegetable or save it for another use, like enriching soup.

Notes: Keep your fingers away from the blades! The Veggetti is known to bite if you're not careful. The best way to keep your fingers safe is to make sure the part of the vegetable you're gripping is dry, unpeeled, and firm. Otherwise use the Veggetti's cap or use a fork to grip the vegetable while you're spiralizing it.

For zucchini, I like to leave the stem on and use it as a grip while spiralizing. I find this to work so well that I never use the Veggetti's cap or a fork when spiralizing zucchini.

For carrots, parsnips, yellow squash, and other vegetables shaped like cones, I like to hold the thin end while spiralizing the thick end so I can use more and waste less of the vegetable.

For eggplant, I like to use the thicker cut because the thinner pasta strands are more fragile than the thicker pasta. Keep in mind that eggplant noodles are notoriously fragile and break easily.

One trick I've learned is to hold the Veggetti a little differently than shown in the manufacturer's instructions. The spiralizing process tends to produce a lot of excess "vegetable" matter and it can get a little messy, with bits of veggie goop falling out the opposite end of the Veggetti and into your plate. I like to cup that end of the Veggetti with my left hand when I spiralize with my right hand. This allows me to catch the vegetable goop in my palm so I can discard it easily.

Best Veggies To Use With The Veggetti:

The Veggetti works best with vegetables that have a tubular shape like zucchini, or cone-like shape like a carrot. The vegetable needs to be able to fit into the blades, and you need to be able to turn the vegetable easily in order to produce nice pasta strands. Therefore, any irregular shaped vegetable, or any oversized or undersized vegetable will not work very well. Use this tool for vegetables sized between 1-1/2" and 2-1/2" diameter. Anything smaller causes too much waste, and anything larger simply cannot fit!

- Zucchini—snip the nose off the zucchini, and use the stem on the other end as a handle to guide the vegetable through the cutter.
- Yellow squash—snip the nose off the squash, and hold the vegetable along the thin end (the stem end) so that the thicker part of the vegetable is turned into noodles and there's less waste.
- Cucumbers—snip the nose off, peel most of the skin but make sure to leave the skin on the gripping end so your hand doesn't slip!
- Carrots, Turnips, and other similar roots—cut ½" from the stem end (the thick end) and grip the thin end. This provides more noodle and less waste. Be careful to choose carrots

that are not cracked, as cracks will cause short circles instead of long strands of pasta.

- Sweet Potatoes, Yams, Potatoes, Beets—if the potato or beet is large, you may need to cut it down to a size that can be handled by the Veggetti. Be VERY careful with these vegetables, they are slippery and can easily cause injury. I always use the Veggetti cap to grip these vegetables while spiralizing.

Worst Veggies To Use With The Veggetti:

- Apples—too large and too difficult to grip.
- Eggplants—too large, and the pasta strands can easily fall apart.
- Vegetables with irregular shapes.

PADERNO-STYLE SPIRALIZERS

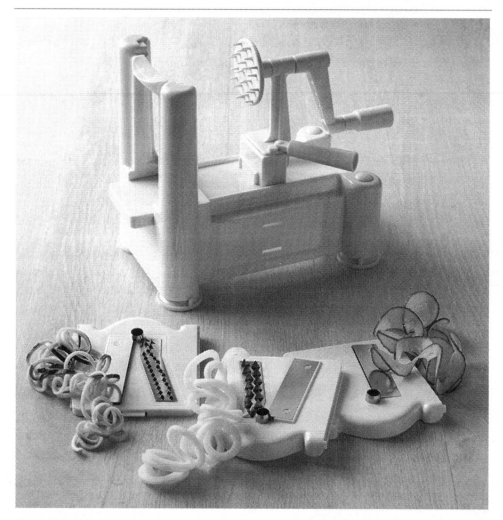

Best for: large quantities of noodles, and greater variety of cuts and shreds. It takes more counter space and more time to set up than a Veggetti, but once it's set up, it works much faster!

The Paderno Spiralizer is a hand-powered tool, which means it is neither battery-powered nor electrical. About the size of a counter-top mixer, it is safer than other hand-held vegetable spiralizers, such as the Veggetti, because the vegetable is inserted into the machine, and directed toward the cutting blades by the action of a turning crank—the cook's hands never get anywhere near the sharp surfaces.

The Paderno has three blades that produce three different types of noodles:

- Thin Spaghetti-sized noodles
- Thick udon/linguini-size noodles
- Wide, flat lasagna noodles—the width depending on the diameter of the vegetable/fruit being cut. This blade also shreds certain vegetables like cabbage, which makes it useful for quickly making slaws and salads.

Here's How To Use The Paderno Safely:

STEP 1: Make certain the machine is firmly "seated" on the counter and that all four suction cups are "engaged." You do this by simply pushing down on the Paderno's legs. Put your body into it! If you don't set the suction cups, as soon as you start using the machine, it will slide right off the counter. To release the suction, simply break the seal by pushing a finger under the suction cups.

STEP 2: Select the appropriate blade depending on how you want to process your vegetable. There are three blades provided with this slicer (thin, thick, and wide).

STEP 3: Sandwich the vegetable to be spiralized or shredded into the machine, holding it in place with the prongs. Be careful to center the vegetable against the blade as well as you can, otherwise it will be more difficult to spiralize.

STEP 4: With your left hand, push the lever forward toward the blade, while turning the crank with your right hand to cut the vegetable. Keep firm pressure against the blade to produce the best results. Do not push on the crank as that might break it. To get shorter "pasta" pieces, cut a groove in the vegetable so that when the "spirals" are sliced off, they are automatically cut, creating the smaller (short) pasta shapes.

Notes: I've found that dense vegetables (such as beets and jicama) can be difficult to successfully spiralize. The Paderno's blades don't always cut deeply enough to slice all the way through, producing full-width noodles that look scored instead of cut. The reason is because dense vegetables require more force to keep them lined up correctly on the blades. But applying too much force to the Paderno can break it. Unfortunately, I haven't found a reliable way to handle this problem other than to grip the lever closer to its hinge and apply more pressure while turning the crank very carefully.

Quirks: Some vegetables may need to be trimmed a bit so that it will easily fit into the center blade.

With some vegetables you'll need to cut a bit off the vegetable so that the crank end will grip it properly. Simply slice off a piece to flatten the end of the vegetable and push the flat end into the prongs to secure it. (With apples, you don't need to do anything except stick the fruit on the crank and start turning.)

Best veggies to use with the Paderno Spiralizer:

The Paderno is particularly good with soft and less dense vegetables and can easily handle larger vegetables that have a diameter of up to 5 inches.

- Apples—particularly nice when cut into the "udon" size
- Cabbages—great for shredding.
- Zucchini—terrific for large zucchini.
- Yellow Squash—also terrific if the squash is large enough.
- Onions—for fast shredding.
- Larger vegetables (up to 5 inches in diameter)

Worst veggies to use with the Paderno spiralizer

- Carrots, Turnips, etc—unless you can find huge carrots or turnips, most carrots are simply too small in diameter to be spiralized by the Paderno. Large carrots also have a tendency to crack on the Paderno. Use a Veggetti or Julienne slicer instead.

- Small zucchini—if your zucchini is less than 1-1/2" in diameter, it will produce more waste than noodles in the Paderno. Use a Veggetti or Julienne slicer instead.
- Any small vegetable or fruit less than 1-1/2" in diameter.

Julienne Slicers & Mandolines

Best for: precision slicing, matchstick cuts, difficult vegetables and fruit, portability.

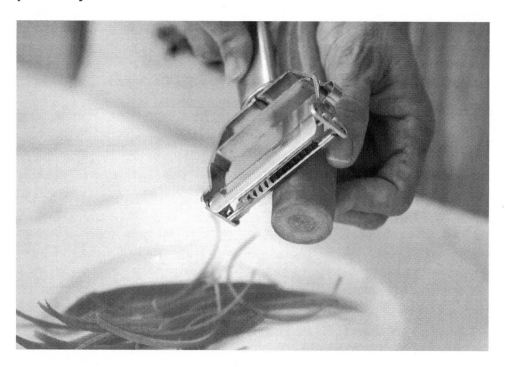

This is the 21st century version of the cooking tool first known as the "mandoline." It is a low-tech tool with no moving parts, just a set of wicked sharp blades that create different sizes and styles of vegetable slices, including crinkle-cut vegetables for "fries."

Best for: nice flat "lasagna" ribbons ranging from thick to ultra-thin, and julienne-cut vegetables

While it is a low-tech gadget, it has been maximized to make it easy to adjust thicknesses while slicing allowing for cuts from paper-thin to thick. There is a purpose-built julienne blade included that will allow for perfect "matchstick" cuts as well. Although the spiralizer-style cutters can create julienne strips, the mandoline is a fast alternative to chopping by hand and is also easier to clean than either the Veggetti or the Paderno style spiralizers.

Best veggies to use with a Mandoline / Julienne Slicer: any!

How To Clean Your Spiralizer

The number one easiest way to clean each of these wonderful spiralizing tools is to wash them under running water immediately after use. If you wash immediately after using, then any vegetable matter will easily slough off of the tool and its blades. Warm soapy water is more effective as it softens the vegetable matter even more. Simply run water over the blades, and use your kitchen brush if needed, then put the tool on your drying rack. The entire process takes 30 seconds.

If you don't clean your spiralizer right away, then you'll have some extra work to do. The entire Veggetti is dishwasher-proof, as are the blades on the Paderno, so for the most part, all you need to do is throw the appliance in the dishwasher and hit "go." But there are times when particles of vegetable matter will cling to the blades. When that happens, there are two easy ways to clean out the debris without putting your fingers at risk.

One method is to use hot water with the sink power sprayer to force the particles out. The second is to use a clean toothbrush to gently scrub the sharp surfaces. (Buy them by the handful at the dollar store and keep a couple in your utensil drawer. You'll be amazed at how useful they'll be.)

For Julienne slicers of any type, hand-washing is recommended. Use the power-rinse at your sink and run hot water through the device to remove any food debris. Wash immediately after use if cutting zucchini or beets, which can leave stains.

5

HOW TO MAKE SPIRALIZED NOODLES & RICE

Just as there are different pasta shapes to fit different dishes (you wouldn't serve a single flabby flat lasagna noodle with sauce poured over it) you can choose specific widths and lengths of spiral-cut vegetables to make your spiralized meal perfect.

CHOOSING THE RIGHT "NOODLE" OR "RICE" FOR THE DISH

Vegetable 'rice" made with a spiralizer can be used interchangeably with rice or couscous in dishes, whether served as a "side" or cooked with other ingredients as part of a more elaborate dish.

Blade Chart
For Paderno and Veggetti-style Spiralizers

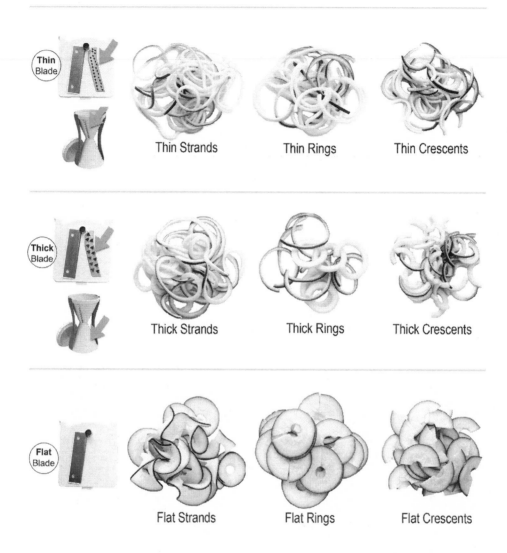

| Thin Strands | Thin Rings | Thin Crescents |

| Thick Strands | Thick Rings | Thick Crescents |

| Flat Strands | Flat Rings | Flat Crescents |

Thick, thin and curly/ring-shaped vegetables strands, however require a little more thought when pairing them up in more complex dishes. Generally speaking, you can use thick and thin vegetable strands in the same way you would use traditional ribbon cut pasta — with thinner strands working best for simple, light sauces such as marinara, and thicker strands for heavier meat sauces.

Spiralized "rings" make an especially fine base for vegetable "pasta" salads. They also work well for some dense vegetables which are difficult to slice into strands, such as potatoes and beets.

Spiralized "crescents" work well with soups, as they can be easer to spoon than rings or strands.

How to Make "Noodles" (Thin, Thick and Flat Strands)

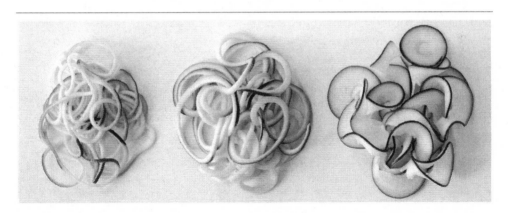

Noodles (strands) are the basic shape produced by spiralizing. If you're spiralizing something, then a long noodle will naturally come out the other end. Simply select your blade according to how thick you want your strands to be.

HOW TO MAKE "RINGS"

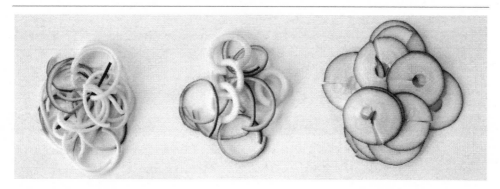

Rings are a little more complex than a simple strand, but still easy to make! Here's how:

Choose an appropriate vegetable. Zucchini, squash, potatoes, beets, cucumber, daikon and large carrots are all good candidates for making rings.

Slit the vegetable along its length on one side. Make sure the slit doesn't reach the center of the vegetable.

Spiralize the vegetable as usual, being careful since the vegetable will be a little weaker than without the slit.

How to Make "Crescents"

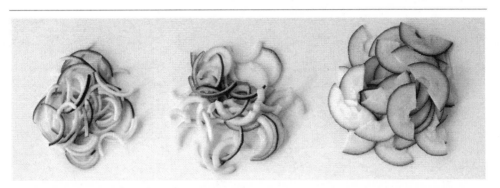

Crescents are a little more difficult because they make the vegetable weak and more difficult to spiralize without breaking. Nevertheless, once you get the hang of it, making crescents is actually easy. Here's how:

Choose an appropriate vegetable. Zucchini, squash, potatoes, beets, cucumber, daikon and large carrots are all good candidates for making rings.

Slit the vegetable along its length on BOTH sides. Here it's extremely important to be careful how deep you make the slits. Try to avoid cutting into the core, as this will cause the vegetable to fall apart while spiralizing.

Spiralize the vegetable carefully.

How to Make "Rice"

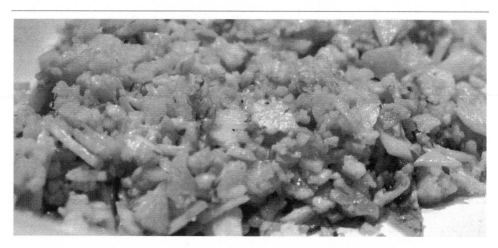

Making "rice" out of cauliflower and broccoli can be a little messy, but it's absolutely delicious and FUN! Here's how:

Choose a small to medium-sized cauliflower. (If you're using broccoli, make sure it's firm and not wilted).

Cut the stem off, you'll be spiralizing the head only.

Use the flat blade on a Paderno-style spiralizer (this method won't work with a Veggetti-style spiralizer).

Spiralize the head of the cauliflower (or broccoli). The resulting chips and grains will be uneven in size, but the unevenness adds a nice texture to a surprising dish.

Cook by boiling or sautéing. Cooked cauliflower (or broccoli) "rice" can be used as a delicious replacement for rice or couscous in just about any dish.

6

HOW TO CHOOSE THE BEST VEGETABLES (AND FRUITS) FOR SPIRALIZING

There's one common-sense rule you need to know when choosing the right vegetable or fruit to slice up. The texture of the fruit or vegetable has to be firm enough to be sliced easily, and the shape needs to be relatively simple and easy to handle.

Spiralizers vary in the size of vegetable or fruit they can accommodate, so look for vegetables that are neither too large nor too small. They should be regular in shape so that the strands come out uniform and don't break. Also, if using fruits, stick to the firmer varieties like apples and pears. Juicy citrus and plush stone fruits simply won't work. But make sure whatever fruit you choose isn't too ripe or the spiralizer will simply turn them to pulp.

VEGETABLE AND FRUITS TO AVOID

Anything that's hollow, like green peppers

Anything that has a tough core, like fresh corn or artichokes

"Stone fruits" like apricots, plums, peaches, and any of the various hybrids

Anything that's too ripe or mushy, like bananas or tomatoes

"Good" Vegetables and Fruits

Generally speaking, root vegetables, squashes, and firm fruits are excellent candidates for spiralizing. Below are the specifics:

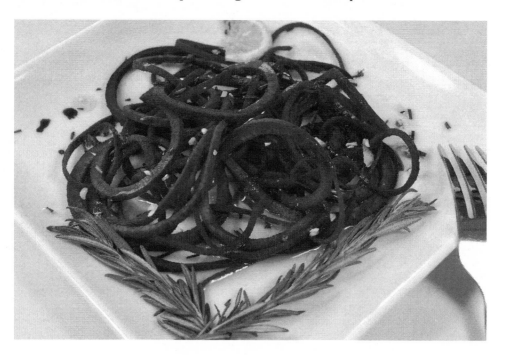

Squashes

Squashes are the go-to vegetables for spiralizer cooking. Whether you choose Italian squash (aka zucchini) or yellow "summer" squash, the result is a mild-tasting, colorful noodle that blends well with any number of other ingredients and spice combinations. These squash are available in supermarkets year round and are always affordable. Leave the skins on but scrub them before spiralizing. It's also useful to chop off the ends so they won't end up going through the blades.

Root Vegetables

Potatoes, turnips, parsnips, sweet potatoes, beets—all the root vegetables are colorful and delicious but they present some special challenges when spiralizing. (See the pro tips for which spiralizers handle carrots best, for instance.)

Miscellaneous Vegetables

If the vegetable is too large to fit the spiralizer comfortably, cut it to fit. With some styles of Spiralizer (like the Paderno type), that's not an issue, but for Veggetti-type spiralizers, best results come from vegetables that are just a little smaller than the circumference of the gadget's opening.

Fruits

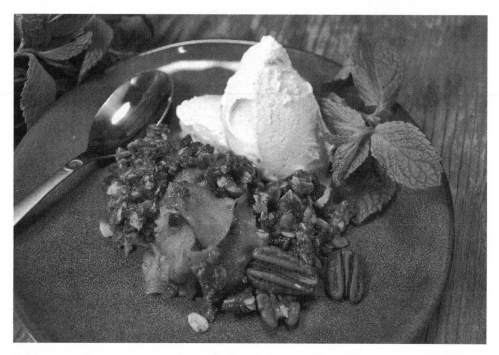

Whatever fruit you use, you'll have an easier time if it's firm. Fair warning: ripe fruits can easily become mushy. Apples are terrific for spiralizing. Pears can work if they're firm. Most other fruits are either too mushy or have pits.

VEGETABLES FOR MAKING "RICE" AND "COUSCOUS"

Canny low-carb cooks have been using "chipped" cauliflower for years as a substitute for rice and potatoes. Spiralizers now make the process easy and a whole lot faster. Broccoli also works really well for this preparation and the smaller "grains" of vegetable add texture and taste (and vitamins) to any dish using rice or grains.

7

8 WAYS TO COOK THE PERFECT SPIRALIZED DISH

There's a reason why neophyte cooks always have some sort of pasta dish in their repertoire—cooking up a filling, flavorful meal that has a pasta base is not much more difficult than boiling water. The good news for health-conscious diners who want to avoid low-quality, high-carb eating is that cooking with spiralized vegetables is just as easy as shaking a box of noodles into a pot of boiling water (and in some cases, even easier!).

RAW

Think outside the pot with your vegetable strands. With just a few exceptions (white potatoes, sweet potatoes), you can eat most vegetables raw, which makes the spiral-cut vegetable strands perfect for a raw food diet in particular. Make spectacular pasta-style salads, and serve them alongside the coleslaw and baked beans at your next barbecue. Create satisfying entrees by topping the raw strands with hot sauces. Just mixing in the sauce will "cook" the strands to al dente perfection.

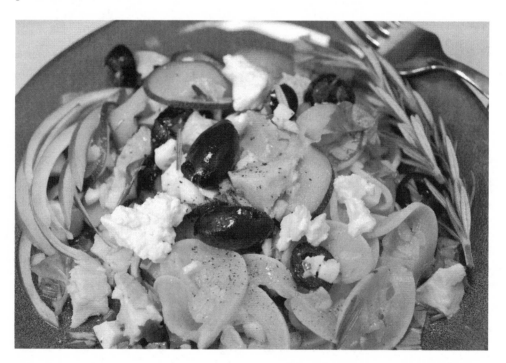

WARM

If you'd rather serve your dish piping hot, you can warm your vegetable strands before adding other ingredients. To do this, simply bring a saucepan of water to a boil, then dump in the raw vegetable strands. Remove after 30 seconds to 1 minutes and drain in a strainer before using.

MICROWAVED

Unlike traditional pasta, which can take on an unpleasant "glue-like" texture when reheated in the microwave, vegetable strands retain their tasty texture. The trick is to mix the sauce in with the vegetable strands before reheating and not to over-nuke the dish. Start with 30-second increments until you find the time that works best.

STEAMED

If you have a steamer or a colander, steaming can be a great way to cook your freshly spiralized noodles while retaining as many nutrients as possible. Steam for 2-5 minutes, depending on the vegetable (potatoes take longer than zucchini). Be careful not to overcook!

BOILED

You might find that some raw vegetables—particularly cruciferous ones like broccoli and cauliflower—need a little bit of cooking to make them more digestible. Simply bring a saucepan of water to boil. Add the vegetable strands and reduce heat to a simmer and cook for 2 to 5 minutes, or until the strands are thoroughly heated. Drain quickly before mixing with other ingredients.

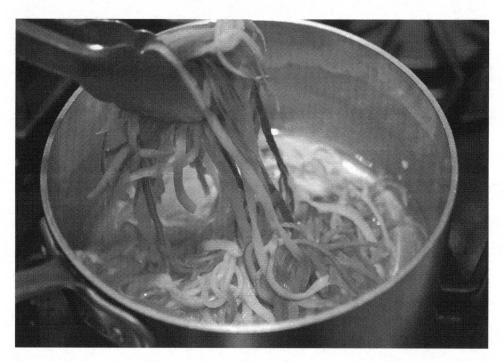

Note: for a nicer texture, try using a very small amount of water (1 inch max) to boil your vegetable noodles. It's ok of there's not enough water to cover the noodles, anything above the water line will steam. After 2-5 minutes, drain the water out of the pot and drizzle some nice extra virgin olive oil over the noodles and a dash of salt. You can use this method with any vegetable anytime — the results are amazing.

SAUTÉED

In this method of cooking, food is cut into small pieces, then browned over medium to high heat. Prior to adding your vegetables, coat the pan with butter, olive oil, coconut oil, or your preferred oil. Generally speaking, the vegetable strands would be added to a sautéed dish at the end, to prevent over-cooking.

STIR-FRIED

Stir-frying is a medium-to-high heat method for quick cooking food in oil, often using a wok. In this method, the food is constantly being stirred to keep the ingredients from sticking or burning. If using vegetable strands made from very dense vegetables (like carrots or broccoli), you might want to steam or lightly boil the vegetables first to quicken the cooking process so that other ingredients don't get over-cooked while the vegetables get tender.

BAKED

Vegetable strands work in any pasta casserole you can imagine, and bake. Simply use as you would any cooked pasta or rice and bake accordingly.

Note: Zucchini and other water-dense vegetables can become very soggy when baked. To minimize sogginess, place freshly spiralized noodles in paper towels for a few minutes to soak up extra moisture.

8

SPIRALIZING TIPS

GENERAL

Spiralizing really is easy once you get the hang of it. Keep these "pro tips" in mind when you're starting out:

- Choose medium-sized zucchini: they're easier to spiralize.
- Don't get too caught up in making "perfect" noodles: a variety of long and short strands actually make the dish more interesting.
- Use only fresh vegetables. Older veggies are too soft and yield poor results, not to mention less nutrition.
- Don't always cook your spiralized noodles! Try them raw, or warm them with the sauce (if a hot dish).
- Make more than you think you need. I'm always amazed at how much shrinkage there is once spiralized zucchini are cooked!

WEIGHT LOSS

If you're interested in weight loss, use these tips to help you adjust your spiralized meals:

- Stick to low-carb toppings for veggie pasta to maximize weight loss.
- Pair vegetable strands with protein for extra satisfaction and satiety.
- Pick nutrient-dense vegetables and fruits to fuel up with fewer calories.
- Add a handful of nuts or seeds to increase fiber, nutrition load, and texture. ·
- Use olive oil, coconut, or nut oils in sauces rather than butter.
- Boost the dish's fiber content by adding vegetables to the sauce.
- Have second helpings if you're still hungry!

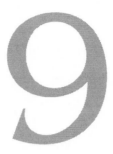

HOW TO USE THIS BOOK

In order to make this book easier to use, we have intentionally condensed the recipe instructions, leaving out repetitive information.

COOKING & SPIRALIZING INSTRUCTIONS

For instructions on how to cook, heat or prepare your spiralized noodles, see Chapter 7.

For help with making strands, rings and crescents out of your favorite vegetables and fruits, see Chapter 5.

RECIPE INGREDIENTS

Unless otherwise noted, when a recipe calls for the following ingredients, you should use:

- Brown sugar—light brown sugar
- Butter—"sweet" (unsalted) butter
- Chicken, beef, or vegetable stock—low-sodium

- Olive oil—extra-virgin

- Salt—sea salt

- Soy sauce—low sodium, tamari-style

- Sugar—white, granulated

- Yogurt—unflavored, unsweetened, Greek-style

RECIPE CONVENTIONS

All spiralized vegetables and fruits appear at the top of ingredients lists.

Most recipes do not suggest how to cook your spiralized vegetable noodles. We leave this up to you. Please refer to Chapter 7 for instructions on how to cook your noodles.

DOWNLOAD THE QUICKSTART GUIDE

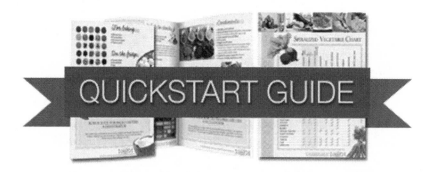

We've found that readers have more success with our book when they use the FREE Quickstart Guide.

Just go to: www.healthyhappyfoodie.org/b1-quickstart

10

SOUPS

"Soup is a lot like a family. Each ingredient enhances the others; each batch has its own characteristics; and it needs time to simmer to reach full flavor."

Marge Kennedy

Asian Pasta with Broth

Prep Time: 15 minutes | Serves: 2

Daikon radishes are rarely used in Western cooking, which is a shame because of its strong peppery flavor that is striking and delicious. This daikon pasta and broth moderates the radish taste with a broth that is just salty enough to cut the heat of the daikon.

Ingredients:

2 large daikon radishes, spiralized

1 cup bok choy, shredded (may substitute spinach)

1 12 oz. block firm tofu, drained and diced

1 Tbsp. dark sesame oil

1/2 cup green onions, sliced (reserve some for garnish)

2 Tbsp. garlic, minced

1 Tbsp. fresh ginger, grated

2 cups chicken broth (preferably low-sodium)

1/2 cup water

1 Tbsp. rice vinegar

2 Tbsp. soy sauce (preferably low-sodium)

Dash of crushed red pepper flakes

Directions:

1. Spiralize the daikon. (Thick rings recommended.).

2. In a small skillet, brown the diced tofu with 1 Tbsp. oil over medium heat.

3. Combine all the ingredients in a medium saucepan and bring to a boil.

4. Cook for 3-5 minutes until the daikon "pasta" is al dente.

5. Garnish with reserved green onion.

Note: for a different flavor, substitute 2-3 Tbsp. of miso paste for the soy sauce.

Nutritional Info: Calories: 663, Sodium: 1,588 mg, Dietary Fiber: 3.2 g,
Total Fat: 15.6 g, Total Carbs: 12.4 g, Protein: 21.6 g

Black Bean & Noodle Soup

Servings: 6 | Prep Time: 25 minutes

This vegetarian dish is healthy, fresh, and quick. You can substitute fresh corn for frozen, if it's in season, which will add additional sweetness and crunch to the dish. If you are not following a vegetarian diet, this soup does well with the addition of shredded chicken or pork. Add the chicken or pork after the broth has simmered for a few minutes, before adding the vegetable noodles.

Ingredients:

2 cups zucchini or yellow squash, spiralized

2 cans (14 oz) vegetable broth

1 jar (16 oz) salsa

1 can (15 oz) black beans, drained and rinsed

2 cups corn kernels (preferably frozen not canned)

Juice of one lime

1/2 Tsp. chili powder

1/2 Tsp. cumin

Fresh cilantro or parsley for garnish

Directions:

1. Spiralize zucchini or squash.

2. Heat the broth to a boil in a medium saucepan.

3. Add the remaining ingredients.

4. Cook for 4-5 minutes, then turn off the heat and add the noodles just before serving.

5.   Garnish with fresh cilantro or parsley and serve hot!

Nutritional Info: Calories: 79, Sodium: 282 mg, Dietary Fiber: 3.7, Total Fat: 0.7 g, Total Carbs: 17.7 g, Protein: 3.4 g

---

BUTTERNUT SQUASH AVOCADO SOUP

Servings: 6 | Prep Time: 30 minutes

This warm filling soup has a lot of potential for customization. Add red pepper flakes for more spice! Replace the water with chicken or vegetable broth for a bit more flavor! Add roasted shredded chicken for a bit of protein! No matter how you make it, the soup is healthy and delicious, great for fighting off winter colds.

Ingredients:

2 cups yellow or butternut squash spiralized

1 large can crushed tomato

3 quarts water

1 Tbsp. vegetable broth

1 large yellow onion, coarsely chopped

1 small can diced green chiles, drained

2 garlic cloves, minced

1 Tsp. cumin

Roasted pumpkin seeds (pepitas)

1 ripe avocado, cubed

1 bunch cilantro, chopped

Fresh cilantro for garnish

Directions:

1. Spiralize squash into thin strands.

2. In a heavy soup pot or Dutch oven, sauté the onion and garlic in the broth until the onion is translucent.

3. Add the crushed tomatoes and water.

4. Stir in the spices and diced chiles.

5. Bring to a boil, reduce heat and simmer for 15 minutes.

6. Return to a boil and add the squash noodles. Cook for 8 minutes or until the vegetable noodles are "done."

7. Serve hot. Garnish with roasted pumpkin seeds, a bit of chopped cilantro, and cubes of ripe avocado.

Nutritional Info: Calories: 79, Sodium: 42 mg, Dietary Fiber: 3.1, Total Fat: 5.0 g, Total Carbs: 9.2 g, Protein: 1.3 g

---

CURRIED LEEK & LENTIL SOUP

Servings: 10 | Prep Time: 30-45 minutes

Using broth instead of water makes this soup more rich and flavorful, but does add extra salt. Use low-sodium broth to reduce that, or replace the broth all together with water. The curry powder can also be increased, for a stronger flavor. You can also substitute yellow or green split peas for the lentils, for a slightly different take on the recipe.

Ingredients:

2 large leeks (white parts only), spiralized

3 large carrots, spiralized

1 yellow onion, coarsely chopped

5 garlic cloves, minced

1/4 Tsp. dried ground ginger, (1 Tbsp. if fresh grated)

2 Tbsp. curry powder (or more, to taste)

1 Tsp. cumin

1 cup green lentils, rinsed

6 cups water OR 6 cups low-sodium chicken broth

3 Tbsp. olive oil

Directions:

1. In a large soup pot, sauté in oil the onion over medium heat until translucent.

2. Spiralize the leeks into strands and add to the soup pot.

3. Sauté until the leeks are tender.

4. Add the spices and stir so the vegetables are evenly coated.

5. Add the lentils and the water or broth.

6. Cover the pot and bring to a boil.

7. Reduce heat and simmer for 25-30 minutes, until lentils are tender. Add additional water or broth, if it seems too dry.

8. 5 minutes before turning off heat, add the spiralized carrots.

9. Serve hot with garnish.

Nutritional Info: Calories: 135, Sodium: 26 mg, Dietary Fiber: 7.4, Total Fat: 4.7 g, Total Carbs: 18.6 g, Protein: 5.8 g

---

Green Chile, Chicken, Squash Soup

Servings: 8 | Cooking time: 90 minutes | Assembly time: 15 minutes

As with any recipe, the better your ingredients the better it will taste. Barbeque your chicken to really punch up the flavor of this healthy hearty soup or roast it with spice rub to add dimension. Either way, the heat and smoke of the peppers contrast nicely with the crunch and freshness of the cabbage, making this dish a healthy and wonderful addition to a menu.

Ingredients:

2 cups yellow squash, spiralized

2 pounds green Poblano chili peppers

1 pound cooked chicken breast, shredded (either roasted or barbecued)

1 medium yellow onion, diced

1 large bunch fresh oregano

6 cups chicken stock

1/2 head of Napa cabbage, shredded

3-4 cloves garlic, peeled

1 lime, cut into wedges

2 Tbsp. chicken broth

Salt and pepper to taste

Directions:

1. Spiralize the squash. (Thick rings recommended.)

2. Roast the Poblano peppers, either over a gas flame, under the oven's broiler, or on the barbeque, turning frequently.

3. When peppers are uniformly blackened, either put in a covered bowl or paper bag to cool.

4. When cool, slip off the blackened skins, remove stems and seeds.

5. In a soup pot, add the onions and broth, then sauté until soft and translucent.

6. Put the onions, garlic, 3 Tbsp. oregano, all the peppers, and 4 cups of chicken stock in a blender. Blend till smooth. (Alternately, put ingredients in a soup pot and use an immersion blender to blend smooth.)

7. Pour the blended mixture into a large soup pot. Add chicken and remaining stock, then simmer for at least 1 hour.

8. If soup seems too thick, add additional stock.

9. Turn off heat and add squash rings.

10. Serve hot, topped with a handful of shredded cabbage, and garnished with oregano and a lime wedge.

Nutritional Info: Calories: 142, Sodium: 955 mg, Dietary Fiber: 1.4, Total Fat: 2.6 g, Total Carbs: 8.9 g, Protein: 20.2 g

Mexican Chicken Noodle Soup

Servings: 6 | Prep Time: 25-30 minutes

A lovely alternative to traditional chicken noodle soup, the jalapeno peppers give a bit of a kick, fresh cilantro adds freshness, and tomatoes give a hint of acidity. This is one of those soups you can cook ahead and refrigerate or freeze, making it excellent for people who are short on time.

Ingredients:

2 cups zucchini, spiralized

6 cups low-sodium chicken stock

2 cans (14 oz) tomatoes, roasted

4 boneless & skinless chicken breasts

5 large garlic cloves, minced

1 yellow onion, chopped

1 large bunch cilantro, chopped (approximately 1 cup)

1 jalapeno pepper, seeded and minced

2 medium carrots, chopped into "coins"

Juice of 2 limes

1 Tsp. cumin

1 Tsp. turmeric

1 Tsp. black pepper

Directions:

1. Spiralize zucchini. (Thin rings recommended.)

2. In a large stock pot heat the onion, carrots, and garlic until the onions are translucent. If it starts to stick, add 1-2 Tsp. water. Add the canned tomatoes (juice and all), the chicken stock and chicken pieces. Bring to a boil until the chicken is cooked through.

3. Remove the chicken from the pot. Set aside to cool.

4. Reduce to a simmer and cover. When the chicken is cool, shred it and return it to the pot along with the noodles, the spices, and lime juice.

5. Continue to simmer for another 30 seconds, then remove from heat.

Nutritional Info: Calories: 149, Sodium: 190 mg, Dietary Fiber: 3.3, Total Fat: 3.0 g, Total Carbs: 10.9 g, Protein: 20.3 g

---

MEXICAN TOMATO SOUP WITH SQUASH NOODLES

Serves: 6 | Prep Time: 30 minutes

This warm filling soup has a lot of potential for customization. Add red pepper flakes for more spice! Replace the water with chicken or vegetable broth for a bit more flavor! Add the roasted and shredded chicken for a bit of protein! No matter how you make it, the soup is healthy, delicious, and great for fighting off winter colds.

Ingredients:

2 cups yellow or butternut squash, spiralized

1 large can crushed tomatoes

3 quarts water

1 Tbsp. vegetable broth

1 large yellow onion, coarsely chopped

1 small can diced green chilies, drained

2 garlic cloves, minced

1 Tsp. cumin

Pumpkin seeds (pepitas), roasted

1 ripe avocado, cubed

1 bunch cilantro, chopped

Directions:

1. Spiralize yellow or butternut squash.

2. In a heavy soup pot or Dutch oven, sauté the onion and garlic until the onion is translucent.

3. Add the crushed tomatoes and water.

4. Stir in the spices and diced chilies.

5. Bring to a boil, reduce heat and simmer for 15 minutes.

6. Turn off the heat and add the squash noodles. Let sit for 1-2 minutes or until the vegetable noodles are done.

7. Serve hot, garnished with roasted pumpkin seeds and a bit of chopped cilantro and cubes of ripe avocado.

Nutritional Info: Calories: 75, Sodium: 51 mg, Dietary Fiber: 2.9 g, Total Fat: 5.0 g, Total Carbs: 6.8 g, Protein: 1.4 g

---

GLUTEN FREE MISO NOODLE SOUP

Servings: 8 | Prep Time: 25-30 minutes

A traditional Japanese dish, this miso soup adds a variety of fresh vegetables to create a healthy, fresh, easy dish. Miso soup is soy based, so if you have soy allergies it's wise to avoid this one, but otherwise, it's considered a great food for people who are ill, especially with the addition of chicken or tofu. Also, if you want a bit more flavor, replace the 3 quarts water with vegetable broth. Be careful this will increase the sodium, however. Be aware that while miso is traditionally made for grains, if you check the ingredients, you can often find ones made with gluten-free grains! Check the label for gluten-containing grains like barley (mugi ortsubu in Japanese), wheat (tsubu), or rye (hadakamugi). Rice (kome or genmai), buckwheat (sobamugi), and millet (kibi) are gluten-free.

Ingredients:

1 cup zucchini, spiralized

4 carrots, spiralized

3 quarts water

2 leeks (white part only), sliced

1 bunch (1/2 pound) Swiss chard (or black kale)

4 carrots, cut into chunks

3 garlic cloves, minced

2 green onions, sliced

1 cup edamame (can use frozen)

1/2 cup gluten-free miso paste

2 Tbsp. water

Optional:

1 package firm tofu, diced into small cubes

1 cup cooked diced chicken

1 cup cooked diced pork

Directions:

1. Spiralize zucchini and carrots.

2. Heat the water in a large stock pot for 1 minute, then add the leeks and garlic. Cook over medium heat for another 5 minutes, stirring occasionally.

3. Separate the chard leaves from the ribs and stalks and set aside. Chop the ribs and stalks, then add to the leek and garlic mixture. Continue to cook until the chard is tender, 8-10 minutes. Stir occasionally so the vegetables don't stick.

4. Add the water to the pot and bring to a boil. Add the chopped carrots and reduce heat to a simmer. Simmer for 5 minutes or until the carrots are almost soft.

5. Chop the chard leaves and add to the soup along with the edamame and spiralized carrots and zucchini. Simmer until the greens wilt, then bring to a boil.

6. Remove 1 cup of boiling water and add it to the miso paste. Add the miso mixture to the soup.

7. If adding optional ingredients, add tofu or pork or chicken now. Cook till heated.

8. Just before serving, add the spiralized noodles.

9. Garnish with sliced green onions.

Nutritional Info: Calories: 137, Sodium: 704 mg, Dietary Fiber: 3.6, Total Fat: 2.3 g, Total Carbs: 20.0 g, Protein: 8.4 g

Pork & Noodle Soup with Greens

Servings: 6 | Prep Time: 25 minutes

Rehydrated mushrooms add umami to any dish, because of the dimension of flavor it creates without adding any unnecessary ingredients. You can adjust the amount of mushrooms you use, depending on your tastes and desires. Don't increase the water just the mushrooms, but remember to drain them well and press on the mushrooms to get out every bit of the soaking liquid to use in your broth!

Ingredients:

4 cups zucchini or yellow squash, spiralized

6 cups chicken broth

1 cup water

3/4 pound pork roast, cut into narrow strips

1 can (8 oz) bamboo shoots, drained

1/4 cup shiitake mushrooms, dried

2 Tbsp. fresh grated ginger

1 small bunch mustard greens, coarsely chopped

1 Tbsp. rice wine (or dry sherry)

1 Tbsp. gluten free soy sauce

Directions:

1. Spiralized zucchini or yellow squash.

2. Pour the cold water over the dried mushrooms and allow to soak for an hour to rehydrate. Drain the mushrooms but save the liquid. Slice the mushrooms thinly discarding the stems.

3. Combine the mushroom soaking water with the broth in a large saucepan and bring to a boil.

4.   Stir in the grated ginger. Cover and reduce heat to a simmer.

5.   Heat 2 Tbsp. of the broth in a heavy (preferably cast iron) skillet. Add the pork and stir fry until no longer pink.

6.   Stir in the rice wine and soy sauce. Cook for another minute, then remove the pork and set aside.

7.   Add another 1 Tbsp. of broth to the wok. Add the mushrooms, mustard greens, and bamboo strips.

8.   Stir-fry for a minute. Stir in the pork and stir-fry for another minute.

9.   Divide the noodles into six bowls. Top the noodles with pork and broth.

Nutritional Info: Calories: 184, Sodium: 935 mg, Dietary Fiber: 1.5, Total Fat: 7.0 g, Total Carbs: 6.6 g, Protein: 22.9 g

---

Pumpkin Noodle Soup

Servings: 6 | Prep Time: 25 minutes

A tiny bit of honey sweetens this dish, without making it over-bearing. It can remain vegetarian (using veggie broth) or be given a bit more richness, by using chicken broth or stock instead. Either way, the longer you cook this soup's base (the pumpkin and broth) the richer the flavor will be. This soup can be modified any number of ways for unique tastes. Try adding a dash of red pepper flakes for more heat, or a half cup of coconut milk for a slightly diet-unfriendly creaminess.

Ingredients:

4 cups pumpkin or squash, spiralized

5 cups vegetable broth

1 large (29-oz.) can pumpkin puree (not the pumpkin, pie filling kind)

1 large yellow onion, diced

1/2 Tbsp. honey

2 Tsp. sage (or 2 Tbsp. fresh sage, chopped)

1 Tsp. cinnamon

1/4 Tsp. ginger

1/4 Tsp. cayenne pepper

1/8 Tsp. nutmeg

Directions:

1. Spiralize the pumpkin or squash.

2. Heat 2 Tbsp. broth in a large saucepot and add the chopped onions. Cook until the onions are translucent, 3-5 minutes. Stir in the spices.

3. Add the pumpkin puree and the rest of the broth. Bring to a boil, then reduce to a simmer.

4.   Stir in the honey.

5.   Add the noodles and simmer for another 2-3 minutes.

Nutritional Info: Calories: 111, Sodium: 647 mg, Dietary Fiber: 6.1, Total Fat: 1.7 g, Total Carbs: 19.8 g, Protein: 6.4 g

---

ROSEMARY ROOT VEGETABLE SOUP

Servings: 6 | Prep Time: 20 minutes

This healthy hearty soup is easy to make and cook while still being rich and satisfying. The root vegetables make it a wintery warm meal that can be served as a first or main course. Try adding other roots vegetables you like, such as celery root. You can also make this recipe vegetarian by substituting vegetable broth.

Ingredients:

3 large parsnips, spiralized

3 large carrots, spiralized

3 large beets, spiralized

1 large yellow onion, sliced

1 quart beef or bone broth

2 quarts water

1 Tbsp. rosemary

1 Tsp. thyme

1 Tsp. oregano

Directions:

1. Spiralize the parsnips, carrots and beets. (Thick rings recommended.)

2. Heat the onions in the bottom of a heavy soup pot or Dutch oven until they are translucent.

3. Add the herbs.

4. Add the broth and water. Bring to a boil.

5. Add the vegetable rings and reduce heat.

6.   Simmer until the "pasta" rings are al dente.

Nutritional Info: Calories: 106, Sodium: 342 mg, Dietary Fiber: 5.9, Total Fat: 0.4 g, Total Carbs: 23.4 g, Protein: 3.5 g

---

Shoyu Cabbage Soup

Servings: 2-3 | Prep time: 30 minutes | Cooking time: 45 minutes

A great first course, this soup is light, delicate, and a little sweet. Using honey instead of sugar changes the nutritional makeup, without removing the hint of sweetness. If the vegetables start to stick to the pan when sautéing, you can add a bit of the vegetable broth to deglaze. If you want to make this soup a little heartier, try adding pre-cooked shrimp or a bit of shredded chicken.

Ingredients:

2 carrots, spiralized

2 zucchini, spiralized

1/2 head Napa cabbage, chopped

1 medium onion, thinly sliced

2 celery stalks, thinly sliced

2 garlic cloves, chopped

4 cups vegetable broth

2 Tbsp. gluten free soy sauce

2 Tbsp. unseasoned rice vinegar

1 Tsp. honey

Hot chili paste and fresh cilantro, for garnish and serving

Directions:

1. Spiralize carrots and zucchini.

2. Add onions, spiral carrots, celery, and garlic to a large pot, and heat to medium. Add 1-2 Tsp. broth if the vegetables stick.

3. Cook until softened, and onions begin to be translucent, about 10 minutes.

4. Add cabbage, broth, soy sauce, vinegar, and honey and bring to a low boil.

5. When boiling, reduce heat and partially cover.

6. Simmer until vegetables are very tender, about 20 minutes.

7. Add spiralized zucchini noodles and cook 3-5 additional minutes till zucchini is softened.

8. Ladle into bowls, and add hot chili paste and cilantro to taste.

Nutritional Info: Calories: 154, Sodium: 1,674 mg, Dietary Fiber: 4.8, Total Fat: 2.4 g, Total Carbs: 22.8 g, Protein: 12.0 g

---

SHRIMP SOUP WITH BOK CHOY

Servings: 8 | Prep Time: 35-45 minutes

This clear soup is rich without being heavy. The use of seafood stock or clam juice gives it a unique flavor, different than most western-inspired soups which clearly demonstrates the Eastern influences. It can be made quickly, making it the perfect conclusion to a long day. Plus you can make the broth ahead, and freeze it, then thaw it out when you're ready to use it. Add the shrimp and noodles, you're on your way to a quick supper!

Ingredients:

3 cups zucchini, spiralized

1 1/2 cups clam juice (or seafood stock)

6 cups chicken stock

2 pounds raw shrimp, cleaned, shelled, and deveined

1 large bok choy, trimmed and sliced thinly

3 green onions, thinly sliced

1 Tbsp. red pepper flakes, crushed

2 Tbsp. ginger, grated

3 large garlic cloves, minced

1/3 pound shiitake mushrooms, sliced

2 Tbsp. water

Directions:

1. Spiralize the zucchini.

2. Heat the water in a large stockpot. Add the bok choy, mushrooms, garlic, ginger, and red pepper flakes. Heat on medium for a minute, then add the broth and clam juice. Cover the pot and bring to a boil.

3. Add the shrimp and sliced green onions. Continue to cook for another 2 minutes or until shrimp are cooked through.

4.   Toss in the noodles. Remove from heat and let stand 5 minutes before serving.

Nutritional Info: Calories: 193, Sodium: 1,385 mg, Dietary Fiber: 0.9, Total Fat: 1.9 g, Total Carbs: 22.3 g, Protein: 25.5 g

---

SIZZLING "RICE" SOUP

Servings: 8 | Prep Time: 25-30 minutes

While you may not get the popping effect of "true" sizzling rice soup, this version is much healthier and just as delicious. Quick frying the cauliflower gives it the crunchiness of the fried rice. You may have to add a little additional oil to fry the cauliflower after frying the shrimp and chicken, but add it slowly because a little goes a long way. This soup also freezes very well.

Ingredients:

2/3 cup cauliflower, spiralized

3 cups chicken broth

1/4 cup baby shrimp, (can use canned or frozen)

1 boneless & skinless chicken breast, cut into bite-sized pieces

2 Tbsp. chopped water chestnuts

1/4 cup bamboo shoots

1/2 cup mushrooms, sliced

1/2 cup bean sprouts

1 large egg .

3 Tbsp. olive oil

1 Tbsp. dry sherry

4 Tbsp. cornstarch

Directions:

1. Spiralize the cauliflower.

2. Combine the egg and cornstarch. Add the shrimp and chicken pieces and stir to coat.

3. Heat 2 Tbsp. oil in a wok.

4. Add the chicken and shrimp. Quickly stir-fry until cooked through. Remove from oil and set aside.

5. In a large saucepan, combine the broth, mushrooms, and bamboo shoots. Bring to a boil.

6. Add the sherry, then reduce heat and simmer.

7. Re-heat the oil in the wok and quickly brown the cauliflower "rice." Remove from oil and drain.

8. Add the "rice" and bean sprouts to the soup and serve immediately.

Nutritional Info: Calories: 135, Sodium: 350 mg, Dietary Fiber: 0.8, Total Fat: 8.1 g, Total Carbs: 7.0 g, Protein: 7.7 g

---

SLOW - COOKER MINESTRONE

Servings: 6 | Prep Time: 6 hours

An easy to make, long-cooking soup, this minestrone does best in a slow cooker left on low. You can add the ingredients: and leave it to simmer all day, without worrying about it. In fact, the longer you cook, the richer the flavors and the more tender the vegetables. Remember NOT to add the greens or veggie spirals until right before serving or they'll get mushy.

Ingredients:

1 cup zucchini or yellow squash, spiralized

4 cups chicken broth (or vegetable broth for a vegetarian soup)

1 can (28 oz) crushed tomato

1 can (15.5 oz.) cannellini beans, drained and rinsed to remove excess salt

1 cup escarole or kale, shredded

2 large carrots, cut into "coins"

2 ribs celery, diced

1 large yellow onion, chopped

3 large garlic cloves, minced

2 Tsp. Italian seasoning

Parsley for garnish

Directions:

1. Spiralize the zucchini or squash. (Thin rings recommended).

2. Combine the broth and canned tomatoes (juice included) with the carrots, celery, garlic, and onion in a slow cooker. Stir in the Italian seasoning. (If using tomatoes that have "Italian seasoning" don't add more.)

3. Cover and cook on low for 4-6 hours, then add the escarole and beans. Cover and increase heat. Cook for another 5-10 minutes, until the greens are wilted.

4. Turn off heat, add the spiralized noodles.

5. Serve hot with parsley garnish.

Nutritional Info: Calories: 60, Sodium: 557 mg, Dietary Fiber: 2.0, Total Fat: 1.5 g, Total Carbs: 7.6 g, Protein: 4.3 g

---

THAI CHICKEN NOODLE SOUP

Servings: 4 | Prep Time: 25-30 minutes

This soup is a delectable, lower-calorie version of Tom Kha Gai, a traditional Thai soup made with lime, fish sauce, and coconut. If you are unable to find shiitake mushrooms, canned straw mushrooms can be easily substituted. Use full-fat coconut milk not light, for the best flavor. Pre-infused broths can also be added to this. Try the kind with lime and chili for extra kick.

Ingredients:

1/2 cup zucchini noodles, spiralized

2 boneless & skinless chicken breasts, cut into bite-size pieces

5 cups chicken broth

1 cup coconut milk

2 jalapeno peppers, seeded and chopped finely

2 large garlic cloves, chopped

1 1/2 inch piece ginger root, grated

1 Tbsp. lime, zest

1/4 cup fresh lime juice

4 Tbsp. fish sauce

2 cups shiitake mushrooms, sliced

2 cups baby spinach leaves

2 Tbsp. cilantro, chopped

Directions:

1. Spiralize the zucchini.

2. Combine the chicken broth, jalapeno, garlic, ginger, lime juice & zest and 3 Tbsp. fish sauce in a medium sauce pan and bring to a simmer.

3. Add the noodles and cook for one minute or until tender. Use tongs to remove the noodles.

4.   Place in a bowl and cover to keep warm.

5.   Add the mushrooms to the broth. Simmer for another four minutes, then add the chicken and the coconut milk.

6.   Continue to simmer until the chicken is cooked through.

7.   Add the spinach and stir until the leaves get limp. Add the chopped cilantro and remaining the Tbsp. of fish sauce.

8.   Divide the cooked noodles into four bowls and pour the soup over the noodles.

Nutritional Info: Calories: 336, Sodium: 8,276 mg, Dietary Fiber: 2.9, Total Fat: 18.7 g, Total Carbs: 23.4 g, Protein: 28.8 g

---

TUNISIAN NOODLE SOUP

Servings: 6 | Prep Time: 25-30 minutes

Tomatoes and hot peppers are staples of Tunisian cooking, which makes this soup both familiar and exotic. Many of the ingredients are used in more familiar cooking, but the way they are combined in this soup gives it an exotic flare.

Ingredients:

2 medium zucchini, spiralized

2 quarts vegetable stock (or chicken stock)

1 pound Swiss chard, chopped coarsely (stems, ribs, and leaves)

1 large red onion, chopped

3 large garlic cloves, minced

2 Tbsp. tomato paste

2 Tbsp. hot pepper sauce

1 Tbsp. fresh lemon juice

Directions:

1. Spiralize the zucchini.

2. Bring the stock to a boil in a stockpot. Add the chard and cook until the chard is wilted.

3. Stir in the tomato paste, hot pepper sauce, garlic, and onion. Return to a boil and then reduce to a simmer.

4. Simmer for 5-10 minutes, then add the noodles. Cook for about 1 minute, or until they are tender.

Nutritional Info: Calories: 137, Sodium: 574 mg, Dietary Fiber: 9.9, Total Fat: 1.4 g, Total Carbs: 29.6 g, Protein: 9.1 g

11

SALADS

"Salad can get a bad rap. People think of bland and watery iceberg lettuce, but in fact, salads are an art form, from the simplest rendition to a colorful kitchen-sink approach."

Marcus Samuelsson

Asian Chicken & Noodle Salad

Servings: 4 | Prep Time: 20 minutes

A delicious cold salad, this recipe uses just a hint of peanut butter to really round out the Asian flavors. Peanut butter is not the most diet-friendly of foods, but in moderation, it can act as a flavor enhancer and really bring out the zest of the other ingredients. Using seasoned rice vinegar can be another trick to amp up the flavor. Brown sugar gives this dish a bit of rich sweetness.

Ingredients:

3 cups zucchini or yellow squash, spiralized

2 cups cooked chicken breasts, cut in bite-size pieces

1/4 cup creamy peanut butter

4 Tbsp. water

5 Tbsp. gluten-free soy sauce

4 Tbsp. rice vinegar

3 Tbsp. chili-garlic sauce

2 Tbsp. fresh ginger, grated

2 Tbsp. brown sugar

1 small bunch cilantro, leaves only chopped

1 bunch green onion, sliced thin

2 medium carrots, grated

1 bell pepper, cut in matchsticks

Directions:

1. Spiralize zucchini or squash.

2. Blanche the noodles if you desire a softer noodle. Otherwise leave raw.

3. In a large serving bowl, combine the noodles, chicken, grated carrots, bell pepper, cilantro, and green onions.

4. In a food processor or blender, combine the peanut butter, soy sauce, chili-garlic sauce, brown sugar, and water. Blend until smooth. If the dressing is too thick, add a little more water.

5. Pour dressing over salad and toss to coat. Chill for an hour.

BEET SALAD

Servings: 2 | Prep Time: 5-10 minutes

A simple classic vinaigrette salad elevates beets to a whole new level. The sweet taste of balsamic vinegar cuts through the tang of the mustard nicely and blends well with the richness of the beets.

Ingredients:

3 beets (about half a pound), spiralized

4 Tbsp. balsamic vinegar

1 Tbsp. Dijon mustard

2 Tbsp. olive oil

1 large garlic clove, minced

2 Tsp. rosemary, minced

Directions:

1. Wash, peel, and spiralize the beets. (Thin strands recommended.)

2. Blanche the noodles if you desire a softer noodle. Otherwise leave raw.

3. Combine the rest of the ingredients and pour over the beets.

4. Toss to coat.

5. Serve immediately.

Nutritional Info: Calories: 204, Sodium: 207 mg, Dietary Fiber: 3.8, Total Fat: 14.8 g, Total Carbs: 16.9 g, Protein: 3.0 g

BEEF SALAD

Servings: 2 | Prep Time: 15 minutes

While one doesn't generally consider something composed largely of roast beef a "salad". This dish is a play on Asian-style beef salads, which has plenty of greens in it. Horseradish takes the place of soy sauce, for that delicious spicy flavor without the high sodium content.

Ingredients:

1 large head of iceberg lettuce, spiralized

1/2 pound rare roast beef, cut into strips

1 basket grape tomato, washed and drained

1 small red onion, thinly sliced

1 large package pre-washed spinach leaves, shredded

2 Tbsp. prepared horseradish (a brand like Trader Joe's without soy, oils, or sugar)

1/4 cup olive oil

1/4 cup beef broth

Directions:

1. Spiralize the iceberg lettuce.

2. Combine the beef, tomatoes, noodles and shredded spinach.

3. Mix the horseradish, olive oil, and beef broth. Pour over the other ingredients.

4. Toss to mix salad.

5. Serve chilled.

Nutritional Info: Calories: 390, Sodium: 1,429 mg, Dietary Fiber: 2.7, Total Fat: 29.4 g, Total Carbs: 10.7 g, Protein: 22.9 g

Light Citrus Ginger Tofu Salad with Carrot and Squash Noodles

Servings: 4 | Prep time: 15 minutes | Cooking time: 20 minutes

This dish is light, bright, and summery. Everything about this dish comes from the complex spices used and the fresh vegetables included. Its vegetarian though can easily be converted to omnivore status by replacing the tofu with sliced chicken or beef.

Ingredients:

For the Salad:

1 large yellow squash, spiralized

3 large carrots, spiralized

Reserved marinade

Zest of 1 lime

Juice of 1/2 lemon

1/8 cup orange juice

3 Tbsp. seasoned rice vinegar

Salt and pepper to taste

1 stalk broccoli - only florets

1 1/2 cup kale, torn off ribs and into bite sized strands

1/2 cup shredded green cabbage

1/3 cup chopped cilantro

1/4 cup basil leaves, chopped

1 Tbsp. sesame seeds, toasted

For the tofu and marinade

1/8 cup orange juice

1/8 cup tamari

1 Tbsp. sesame oil

1 Tsp. fresh ginger, finely grated

1 garlic clove, finely minced

2 Tsp. real maple syrup

1/4 Tsp. cayenne pepper

1 package extra firm tofu

Directions:

Tofu and Marinade:

1. Preheat oven to 350° F.

2. In a large bowl, mix together orange juice, tamari, sesame oil, ginger, garlic, maple syrup, and cayenne. Set aside.

3. Cut tofu into 1 inch cubes and put into a baking pan with 1/4 inch space between.

4. Pour the marinade over the tofu.

5. Bake tofu for 15 minutes.

6. Stir.

7. Bake for 15 more minutes.

8. Take tofu pieces out and place on a plate to drain and cool.

9. Pour off remaining marinade and set aside.

Salad and Dressing:

1. Spiralize the carrots and squash. (Thin strands recommended.)

2. Heat a pot of water to boiling, and blanch squash and carrots until just tender, but still al dente.

3. Drain well, and set aside.

4. Take remaining marinade and add lime zest, lemon juice, orange juice, vinegar, and maple syrup. Add sea salt and pepper to taste, set aside.

5. Bring another pot of water to a bowl, blanch the broccoli florets for 30 seconds – 1 minute depending on the desired degree of crispness.

6. Remove and rinse with cold water, drain well.

7. Put broccoli, carrot, squash, cabbage, kale, cilantro, basil, and sesame seeds in a large bowl and toss.

8. Take dressing that had been set aside and toss over salad till well coated.

9. Put the salad on a serving dish or in a serving bowl and top with drained cooled tofu and garnish with additional sesame seeds.

Nutritional Info: Calories: 154, Sodium: 618 mg, Dietary Fiber: 4.3, Total Fat: 6.2 g, Total Carbs: 20.6 g, Protein: 7.2 g

Colorful Carrot & Beet Slaw

Servings: 4 | Prep Time: 15 minutes

A quick to whip up, delicious and bright dish. The vinaigrette relies on old standards — Dijon mustard and vinegar without using the traditional olive oil. If you want to change up the flavors without losing the dish's substance, try using pickled beets instead of traditional ones. This will give the salad a bit more tangy flavor while retaining all the crunch of fresh beets.

Ingredients:

3 large beets, spiralized

4 large carrots, spiralized

3 Tbsp. Dijon mustard

4 Tbsp. red wine vinegar

4 Tbsp. olive oil

1 Tsp. black pepper

Parsley for garnish

Directions:

1. Spiralize carrots and beets. (Thin strands recommended.)

2. Blanche the noodles if you desire a softer noodle. Otherwise leave raw.

3. Place beet and carrot noodles into a plate.

4. Combine oil, vinegar, mustard, and pepper, whisk well.

5. Pour vinaigrette over noodles. Garnish with parsley.

Nutritional Info: Calories: 202, Sodium: 370 mg, Dietary Fiber: 3.2, Total Fat: 14.1 g, Total Carbs: 14.2 g, Protein: 1.7 g

Greek Pasta Salad

Servings: 6 | Prep Time: 15 minutes

Generally, one thinks of Greek salads as either mixtures of tomatoes and cucumbers doused in oil, or cold-cut heavy pasta concoctions. This salad is neither, but the unmistakable Greek flavor comes through. You can also throw in more spices, or different vegetables to suit. We recommend adding a bit of flat Udon cut cucumber as well, to really jazz up the dish.

Ingredients:

4 medium zucchini, spiralized

1 bunch green onions, sliced

1 basket cherry tomatoes, halved

1 (27-ounces) package sliced white mushrooms

1 large bell pepper, seeded and sliced into matchsticks

1 4 can oz. can pitted black, olives, drained

1 cup feta cheese, crumbled

2 large garlic cloves, minced

2 Tsp. basil

1 1/2 Tsp. oregano

1/2 Tsp. black pepper

4 Tbsp. olive oil

1/2 cup red wine vinegar

Directions:

1. Spiralize zucchini. (Thick rings recommended.)

2. Blanche the noodles if you desire a softer noodle. Otherwise leave raw.

3. In a large bowl combine the oil, vinegar, garlic, basil, oregano, and pepper. Whisk to blend.

4. Add remaining ingredients including noodles, and toss to distribute dressing evenly.

5. Chill overnight to blend flavors.

Nutritional Info: Calories: 291, Sodium: 366 mg, Dietary Fiber: 6.7, Total Fat: 14.9 g, Total Carbs: 23.7 g, Protein: 19.3 g

---

Mediterranean Pasta Salad

Servings: 4 | Prep Time: 12 minutes

This "pasta" salad with vinaigrette is an excellent accompaniment for a Greek feast! Pair it with lamb or pork, especially in a vinegar-based marinade as a delicious side dish. For an even more Mediterranean flair, substitute Kalamata olives for the black olives, but be aware how salty they are!

Ingredients:

---

4 medium zucchini, spiralized

2 cups cooked chicken breasts, cut in bite-sized pieces

3 hard-boiled egg whites, diced

1 small red onion, diced

2 garlic cloves, minced

3 Tbsp. olive oil

Juice of 1/2 lemon

1 Tsp. basil

1/2 Tsp. dried rosemary

Sliced black olives (for garnish)

Directions:

---

1. Spiralize the zucchini.

2. Blanche the noodles if you desire a softer noodle. Otherwise leave raw.

3. Combine the noodles, chicken, diced egg whites, and red onion in a small bowl.

4. Combine the other ingredients and whisk to blend well. Pour over the noodle/chicken mixture and toss to blend.

5. Garnish with sliced olives if desired.

Nutritional Info: Calories: 215, Sodium: 91 mg, Dietary Fiber: 2.7, Total Fat: 13.1 g, Total Carbs: 9.0 g, Protein: 17.9 g

---

NOODLES & HUMUS SALAD

Servings: 4 | Prep Time: 10 minutes

Hummus, made from mashed chickpeas is known for a creamy, delicious flavor. This salad taps into that creaminess to create a rich savory dressing with very little additional fats or oils. The sesame oil is largely for flavoring, and can be left out, as desired. Try experimenting with different kinds of hummus. Red pepper hummus or garlic flavored might add kick!

Ingredients:

4 cups zucchini, spiralized

2 medium carrots, spiralized

3/4 cup prepared hummus

1 bell pepper, seeded and diced

3 green onions, thinly sliced

1 Tbsp. dark sesame oil (if desired)

4 Tbsp. gluten free soy sauce

4 Tbsp. rice vinegar

1 Tsp. ginger

2 Tbsp. fresh mint

1 Tsp. crushed red pepper flakes

Directions:

1. Spiralize the zucchini and carrots. (Thin crescents recommended.)

2. Blanch the carrot noodles. If you like soft zucchini noodles, then blanch the zucchini, otherwise leave uncooked.

3. Combine the noodles with the peppers and green onions in a large bowl.

4. Combine the oil, vinegar, herbs, and spices.

5. Using a food processor, mix the spice mixture into the hummus and blend until smooth.

6. Mix well and pour over the noodle/vegetable combination.

Nutritional Info: Calories: 176, Sodium: 917 mg, Dietary Fiber: 4.9, Total Fat: 7.6 g, Total Carbs: 20.3 g, Protein: 5.5 g

ONE POT KALE AND CAULIFLOWER PILAF

Servings: 2-4 | Cooking time: 30 minutes | Assembly time: 10 minutes

Kale is considered one of the newest super foods. This mix of kale and cauliflower is nutty, delicious, and fresh with the creamy inclusion of goat cheese. Feel free to try different kinds of savory goat cheese from herb-flavored to garlic-flavored. Toasting the cauliflower really brings out the taste, without adding too many complicated steps to the recipe.

Ingredients:

2/3 cup cauliflower, spiralized

1 bunch kale, washed and chopped into bite-sized pieces

1 lemon, zested and juiced

2 scallions, finely minced

3 Tbsp. toasted pine nuts

2 Tbsp. olive oil

1/4 cup crumbled goat cheese

Salt and pepper to taste

Directions:

Cauliflower:

1. Spiralize cauliflower.

2. Heat a large skillet on medium-high.

3. Add cauliflower and sauté until just turning brown then remove from heat. About 5-8 minutes.

4. Kale:

5. Put a steamer in a large pan, fill pan with 1/2 inch water. Add Kale to steamer.

6. Cover and steam for 3-5 minutes until wilted but not soft.

102

Assembling the dish:

1. In a large serving bowl, combine half of lemon juice, lemon zest, scallions, pine nuts, and goat cheese.

2. Toss kale, cauliflower, and above mixture together.

3. Serve immediately.

Nutritional Info: Calories: 118, Sodium: 9 mg, Dietary Fiber: 1.1, Total Fat: 11.5 g, Total Carbs: 4.5 g, Protein: 1.7 g

---

Pasta Primavera Salad

Servings: 4 | Prep Time: 15 minutes

Vinaigrette are a delicious way to season salads without a lot of effort. This recipe relies instead on the flavors of the garlic and Italian seasoning to make it tasty. If you want a bit more zing, add a dash of red pepper flakes for a bit of spice.

Ingredients:

4 cups zucchini or yellow squash, spiralized

2 large carrots, spiralized

1 bell pepper (any color), diced

1 bunch green onions, chopped

6 Roma tomatoes, seeded and diced

5 Tbsp. olive oil

1/2 cup red wine vinegar

1-2 Tsp. garlic, minced

1 Tbsp. Italian seasoning

Parmesan cheese

Dash of black pepper

Parmesan cheese for garnish

Directions:

1. Spiralize the zucchini or squash and carrots.

2. Blanche the carrots and squash if a softer noodle is desired. Otherwise leave raw.

3. Combine chopped vegetables with the warm pasta.

4. Mix olive oil, vinegar, garlic, and Italian seasoning.

5. Add black pepper to taste.

6. Toss pasta to combine ingredients.

7.   Garnish with a sprinkle of Parmesan cheese.

Nutritional Info: Calories: 280, Sodium: 47 mg, Dietary Fiber: 4.2, Total Fat: 20.2 g, Total Carbs: 21.3 g, Protein: 3.6 g

---

ROASTED BABY TURNIPS WITH DIJON-SHALLOT VINAIGRETTE AND BEET NOODLES

Servings: 4-6 | Cooking time: 30 minutes | Assembly time: 10 minutes

Roasting the turnips in mustard really enhances their flavor. Try tossing the beet noodles in a little of the dressing before serving, if you want a stronger mustard flavor. You can also garnish with caramelized shallots if you want a bit more tang.

Ingredients:

1 bunch red beets, peeled and spiralized

2 bunches baby turnips, peeled and chopped into quarters

Salt and pepper to taste

2 Tbsp. white wine vinegar

2 Tbsp. Dijon mustard, divided

2 Tbsp. olive oil

4 Tbsp. vegetable broth

1 shallot, finely minced

Salt and pepper to taste

1 Tbsp. tarragon, chopped

Directions:

Turnips:

1. Preheat oven to 400° F.

2. Toss turnips with 1 Tbsp. mustard, salt and pepper.

3. Spread in a single layer on a baking sheet and bake 10-15 minutes, or until softened inside, slightly brown and caramelized outside.

Beets:

1. Spiralize the beets. (Thick crescents recommended.)

2. Boil a pot of lightly salted water.

3. Add spiral cut beets and blanch until just soft 5-7 minutes.

4. Drain and set aside.

Dressing:

1. Either using a blender or a hand whisk, whisk together vinegar, broth, and remaining mustard.

2. Slowly add the olive oil in a thin stream and whisk till emulsified.

3. Whisk in shallots.

Assembling the dish:

1. Toss the turnips with the dressing.

2. Plate on a bed of beet noodles.

3. Serve at room temperature.

Nutritional Info: Calories: 68, Sodium: 143 mg, Dietary Fiber: 1.2, Total Fat: 5.0 g, Total Carbs: 5.3 g, Protein: 1.0 g

SHAVED ASPARAGUS, YELLOW SQUASH, AND MINT SALAD

Servings: 4 | Cooking time: 10 minutes | Assembly time: 10 minutes

Using sunflower seeds are a fun addition to this recipe that changes the taste, without adding much expense or difficulty in getting ingredients. Asparagus is generally cooked far too thoroughly; making the fact that it is used raw here is quite unique in both technique and taste. The olive oil can be replaced with avocado or coconut oil to slightly change the nutrition profile and taste, as desired.

Ingredients:

1 large yellow squash, spiralized

1 bunch asparagus

1 Tbsp. mint, chopped

3 Tbsp. lemon juice

3 Tbsp. sherry or white wine vinegar

1 Tsp. honey

1 Tbsp. extra virgin olive oil

1/4 cup sunflower seeds

Directions:

Dressing:

1. In a medium sized bowl, whisk together lemon juice, vinegar, honey, and olive oil. Set aside.

Salad:

1. Spiralize yellow squash. (Thin strands recommended.)

2. Heat a pot of lightly salted water to boiling.

3. Add squash and blanch till just tender, but still al dente, about 2 minutes.

4. Drain well, and allow to cool fully.

5. Using a vegetable peeler, shave the asparagus very thinly lengthwise. Shavings should be very thin.

6. Toss asparagus, cooled squash noodles, and mint together

7. Toss asparagus mixture with dressing.

8. Add salt and pepper to taste.

9. Sprinkle with sunflower seeds.

Nutritional Info: Calories: 119, Sodium: 12 mg, Dietary Fiber: 2.0, Total Fat: 5.3 g, Total Carbs: 6.8 g, Protein: 2.5 g

---

VEGETABLES WITH ROSEMARY VINAIGRETTE

Servings: 10 | Prep Time: 40 minutes

As you'll see in our alternate instructions, this dish works well as either a sauté or a bake. Either way, we don't use oil to cook the vegetables in but stick to vegetable broth. Be aware this adds salt to the dish so if you're seasoning it with additional salt, use a careful hand. You can always increase the balsamic vinegar if you want a bit sweeter a flavor.

Ingredients:

4 carrots, spiralized

2 turnips, spiralized

4 yellow squash, spiralized

2 medium sweet potatoes, spiralized

2 bell peppers, de-seeded and julienne sliced

1 large yellow onion, thinly sliced

1 bunch fresh rosemary, coarsely chopped

4 leaves fresh sage, chopped (or 1 Tsp. dried sage)

1 Tbsp. Italian seasoning

3 large garlic cloves, minced

3 Tbsp. balsamic vinegar

1 Tsp. black pepper

3 Tbsp. vegetable broth

Directions:

1.   Spiralize the carrots, turnips, squash, and sweet potatoes.

2.   Heat the broth in a large skillet and sauté the vegetables until they are crisp/tender.

3.   Combine the vinegar and remaining ingredients and pour over the vegetables in the skillet.

4.   Cook for another 5 minutes to blend flavors.

Note: A variation on this dish is roasted vegetables with rosemary vinaigrette. Place all the vegetables in a large baking pan. Combine the oil, vinegar, and spices as if for salad dressing. Pour over the vegetables and bake for an hour at 400° F or until the vegetables are tender.

Nutritional Info: Calories: 69, Sodium: 63 mg, Dietary Fiber: 2.7, Total Fat: 0.5 g, Total Carbs: 14.5 g, Protein: 1.3 g

---

Zucchini and Squash Summer Salad with Golden Raisins, Pistachios, and Mint

Servings: 4 | Prep time: 15 minutes | Cooking time: 20 minutes

A delicious summery salad that pairs well with chicken. The vegetable stock adds a dimension to the noodles that plain water cannot, while adding no fat to the dish. Excellent for serving to vegetarians, there's no need for meat to make this dish delicious, but if you want to serve it as a main course, try topping with a grilled chicken breast.

Ingredients:

1 large yellow squash, spiralized	1 1/4 cup vegetable stock
1 large zucchini, spiralized	1 medium shallot, finely chopped
1 Tbsp. lemon zest	1/2 cup golden raisins
Juice of 1 lemon	1/4 cup pistachios, chopped
1/2 Tsp. honey	2 Tbsp. fresh mint, chopped
3 garlic cloves, crushed	Salt and pepper to taste

Directions:

Noodles:

1. Spiralize the yellow squash and zucchini.
2. Bring the vegetable stock to a boil.
3. Add spiralized vegetables. Boil for 1-2 minutes until just tender.
4. Drain reserving the broth. Set aside to cool.

Dressing:

1. Whisk together lemon zest, lemon juice, honey, and 1/4 cup reserved broth.

2. Add garlic cloves and set aside for at least 30 minutes.

Assembling the dish:

1. Heat a large skillet to medium heat.

2. Add shallots, raisins, pistachios and 1/2 - 1 Tsp. salt.

3. Toss well and cook 1-2 minutes till lightly toasted. If mixture sticks to pan, add 1-2 Tsp. reserved broth.

4. Add cooked noodles, and cook 2-3 more minutes till slightly crispy and golden.

5. Remove the garlic cloves from the dressing.

6. Toss dressing with noodle mixture.

7. Sprinkle with chopped mint.

8. Serve at room temperature.

Nutritional Info: Calories: 139, Sodium: 32 mg, Dietary Fiber: 3.8, Total Fat: 4.0 g, Total Carbs: 25.7 g, Protein: 4.7 g

---

Zucchini, Squash, and Spinach Salad with Apples and Cranberries

Servings: 4 | Cooking time: 30 minutes | Assembly time: 15 minutes

High in vitamins, fiber, and micronutrients, spinach is one of nature's superfoods. This salad couples excellent fresh flavors with vegetables packed with beneficial nutrients. Plus it tastes great! The sweetness of the apples blends well with the stronger flavor of the zucchini and squash. Everything suits perfectly with the heartiness of the spinach. Remember though to rinse your spinach well!

Ingredients:

2 large zucchinis, spiralized

2 large yellow squashes, spiralized

1 apple (gala or Fuji recommended), spiralized

1 bunch baby spinach

1 small onion, finely diced

1 bunch green onions, chopped (green parts only)

1/2 cup cranberries, finely chopped

1 bunch flat-leaf parsley, finely chopped

1 large lemon, juiced

Directions:

1. Spiralize zucchini and squash. (Thin strands recommended.)

2. Blanche the zucchini and squash if a softer noodle is desired. Otherwise leave raw.

3. Spiralize apple (thin strands recommended). Toss apple strands with lemon juice to prevent browning and add flavor. Set aside.

4. Heat a heavy bottomed skillet to medium

5. Add chopped onion and celery, then cook till softened, approximately 5-8 minutes. Do not let them brown, just wilt and soften. If they start to stick, add 1-2 Tsp. water.

6. Add salt and pepper to taste.

7. Set aside to cool.

8. Add cranberries, green onions, and parsley to the cooked celery and onions.

9. Add vegetable noodles and apple.

10. Add salt and pepper, and additional lemon juice to taste.

11. Refrigerate for at least 20 minutes prior to serving.

12. Just before serving, toss noodle mixture with spinach.

13. Serve cool or cold.

Nutritional Info: Calories: 102, Sodium: 104 mg, Dietary Fiber: 7.2, Total Fat: 0.9 g, Total Carbs: 21.9 g, Protein: 5.9 g

---

SOUTH OF THE BORDER JICAMA-AVOCADO SALAD

Servings: 2 | Prep Time: 5-10 minutes

One of the latest and greatest wonder foods, avocados is packed with healthy fats and lots of flavor. Just 1/2 an avocado is enough to flavor a whole salad and give you your daily dose of Omega-3s without breaking your diet. Jicama's fresh taste and crunchy texture blends well with the creaminess of the avocado.

Ingredients:

2 medium jicama, spiralized

3 limes, juiced (about 1/4 cup)

1/2 avocado, mashed

1/2 Tsp. chili powder

1 large garlic clove, minced

Dash of red pepper flakes (optional)

Directions:

1. Remove the jicama's papery outer "skin" and spiralize. (Thin strands recommended.)

2. Set aside in a medium bowl.

3. Mix other ingredients well, then mix in jicama.

4. Serve immediately.

Nutritional Info: Calories: 182, Sodium: 12 mg, Dietary Fiber: 12.4, Total Fat: 10.1 g, Total Carbs: 26.8 g, Protein: 2.8 g

DILL SALMON PASTA SALAD

Servings: 6 | Prep Time: 20 minutes

A take on a version of traditional tea sandwiches, this pasta uses a hint of sour cream to mimic the cream cheese. The red wine vinegar brightens the dish, making it a little bit more tangy, tart, and savory. The zucchini pasta keeps things light and delicious, without all the carbs of traditional pasta.

Ingredients:

4 large zucchini, spiralized

1 can (15 oz) salmon, drained and flaked

1 bunch fresh dill, minced

2 bell peppers, seeded and minced (can use any color)

1/3 cup vegetable broth

1 Tbsp. olive oil

1/3 cup Dijon mustard

1/2 red wine vinegar

2 garlic cloves, minced

Directions:

1. Spiralize zucchini.

2. Blanche the zucchini noodles if a soft noodle is desired, otherwise leave uncooked.

3. Whisk the olive oil with the mustard, garlic, broth, and vinegar in a large bowl.

4. Add the noodles, peppers, and salmon.

5. Toss to combine.

Nutritional Info: Calories: 93, Sodium: 227 mg, Dietary Fiber: 3.7, Total Fat: 4.8 g, Total Carbs: 11.1 g, Protein: 4.2 g

Thai Green Papaya Salad

Servings: 4 | Prep Time: 20-25 minutes

In Thai cooking, green papaya is considered one of the most healthful foods available. Considered by some as a detoxifying agent, it not only has a number of benefits but also tastes great. This salad mixes traditional Thai flavors with fresh ingredients, making it an excellent addition to any meal, especially one with other Thai flavors.

Ingredients:

2 green papayas, peeled and spiralized

2 medium carrots, spiralized

2 cups bean sprouts

10 grape tomatoes, cut in half

1/2 cup fresh basil, chopped roughly

1/2 cup unsalted peanuts, chopped coarsely

1/2 Tsp. gluten free soy sauce

2 Tbsp. fish sauce

Juice of two limes

Directions:

1. Spiralize the papaya and carrots.

2. Mix the papaya, carrots, tomatoes, and chopped basil.

3. Combine the oil, soy sauce, fish sauce, and lime juice. Pour the dressing over the salad. Toss to combine.

4. Garnish with chopped peanuts.

Nutritional Info: Calories: 265, Sodium: 3680 mg, Dietary Fiber: 4.8, Total Fat: 13.5 g, Total Carbs: 35.7 g, Protein: 13.8 g

12

SIDES

"You don't have to cook fancy or complicated masterpieces - just good food from fresh ingredients."

Julia Child

POTATO-VEGGIE LATKES

Servings: 6 | Prep Time: 20 minutes

These delicious fried crispy morsels are easy and quick to whip up. Fried in oil, it should be left to drain well before eating to get excess grease off but taste best piping hot. Pair them with sour cream or applesauce for a homey hearty side dish.

Ingredients:

4 large baking potatoes, spiralized

1 large carrot, spiralized

1 large yellow onion, grated

2 eggs, beaten

3 Tbsp. almond flour or cornstarch

Dash of kosher salt

Dash of black pepper

Vegetable oil for frying

Directions:

1. Spiralize carrot and potatoes. (Thick rings recommended.)

2. Combine in with the grated onion in a colander set over a large bowl. Press down with the back of a spoon to squeeze as much moisture as possible out of the mixture.

3. Let drain for five minutes.

4. Discard the liquid, then combine the vegetables with eggs and almond flour.

5. Add ground pepper and salt.

6. Heat oil in a low frying pan till just sizzling.

7. Using a spoon, drop dollops onto the baking pan and flatten with the back of a spoon or spatula.

8. Fry approximately 5 minutes on one side, then flip. Pancake should be crispy and golden brown.

Nutritional Info: Calories: 235, Sodium: 67 mg, Dietary Fiber: 4.8, Total Fat: 1.6 g, Total Carbs: 50.1 g, Protein: 6.2 g

---

BAKED ZUCCHINI AND POTATO PANCAKES

Servings: 2 | Prep time: 10 minutes | Cooking time: 25 minutes

Most vegetable pancakes are fried in butter, which while delicious is hardly diet-friendly. These crispy rich pancakes are oven-baked dramatically reducing the fat content. This recipe uses no added oils and only a bit of cooking spray on the pan and there is no messy high-calorie frying. Try adjusting the cooking time till you get the degree of crispiness you like. Using almond flour adds nuttiness to the pancakes, but cornstarch works just as well.

Ingredients:

2 cups zucchini, spiralized

1/2 cup potato, spiralized

Salt and pepper to taste

1 egg

1 Tbsp. chopped parsley

1 Tsp. lemon zest

1-2 Tsp. almond flour, cornstarch, or potato starch

Directions:

1. Preheat oven to 350° F.

2. Spiralize the zucchini and potato. (Thick rings recommended.)

3. Let stand in a colander for at least 30 minutes to drain. The better drained they are, the better the pancakes will stick together.

4. In a bowl beat egg, parsley, and lemon zest. Add a pinch of salt and pepper and beat well.

5. Take zucchini and potato mixture out of the colander and roll in paper towels. Squeeze well to drain all residual moisture.

6. Add 1-2 Tsp. almond flour, cornstarch, or potato starch to soak up the last of the moisture.

7. Mix zucchini and potato mixture with egg mixture and toss well to coat.

8. Spray a large glass baking dish with cooking spray.

9. Place dollops of mixture (approx 2 Tbsp.) in dish with space between them. Take a spatula and press down lightly to flatten.

10. Bake approximately 8 minutes, till lightly browned on bottom then flip over and bake an additional 5 minutes till fully browned.

11. Serve immediately.

Nutritional Info: Calories: 222, Sodium: 56 mg, Dietary Fiber: 6.8 g, Total Fat: 9.3 g, Total Carbs: 27.7 g, Protein: 11.6 g

CABBAGE AND APPLE SAUTÉ

Servings: 4 | Prep Time: 30 minutes

The combination of bacon, apples, and cabbage is a classic and delicious one. With its slightly German feel, this recipe makes an excellent side dish for pork roast, but can also be served alongside other main dishes

Ingredients:

2 tart apples, spiralized

1/2 pound bacon

1 medium cabbage head, spiralized

1 large yellow onion, coarsely chopped

1 cup water

1-2 Tbsp. lemon juice

1 small bay leaf

Freshly ground pepper

Directions:

1. Fry bacon until crisp.

2. Drain all but 2 Tbsp. bacon fat.

3. Spiralize the cabbage.

4. Place the chopped onion in the skillet.

5. Stirring frequently, cook onions until they are translucent, being careful not to let them stick to the pan.

6. Add the cabbage and bay leaf.

7. Cover and reduce heat.

8. Simmer for 20-30 minutes until the cabbage is tender but still a bit crisp.

9.   While simmering the cabbage, spiralize the apples into strands. Squeeze 1-2 Tbsp. of fresh lemon juice over the apple spirals. Set aside.

10. When the cabbage is ready, remove bay leaf and mix in the apple noodles.

11. Place the hot mixture in dish and garnish with bacon.

12. There's no need to add salt to this dish; the bacon fat will supply plenty of sodium.

Nutritional Info: Calories: 374, Sodium: 1,318 mg, Dietary Fiber: 4.4, Total Fat: 23.8 g, Total Carbs: 17.4 g, Protein: 21.6 g

---

CURRIED VEGETABLE COUSCOUS

Servings: 2 | Prep Time: 15 minutes

An excellent healthy vegetarian side dish, the complexity of the spices gives it such flavor and depth that you won't even notice it's low fat! Substituting cauliflower for traditional couscous adds nutrients, reduces carbs, and keeps the dish light and fresh. Remember to drain and rinse the chickpeas well to remove excess salt from the dish.

Ingredients:

1/2 cup cauliflower heads, spiralized

3 Tsp. olive oil

1 green onion, sliced (green tops included)

1/2 bell pepper, diced

1 small yellow squash, diced

1 ripe Roma tomato, chopped

3/4 cup canned chickpeas (rinse and drain to remove salty liquid)

1 garlic clove, minced

1 Tsp. curry powder

1/4 Tsp. ginger

1/4 Tsp. cumin

1/4 Tsp. cinnamon

1/4 Tsp. cayenne pepper (leave out if using madras-style curry powder)

Parsley for garnish

Directions:

1. Spiralize the cauliflower to make "couscous."

2. Sauté the garlic, onion, and spices until the onion is translucent.

3. If onions begin to stick, use 1-2 Tsp. of water to release them.

4. Add the vegetables, chickpeas and cauliflower couscous, and sauté for another five minutes.

5. Turn off the heat and let sit to combine flavors.

6. Serve hot with parsley garnish.

Nutritional Info: Calories: 389, Sodium: 43 mg, Dietary Fiber: 16.8, Total Fat: 12.3 g, Total Carbs: 57.4 g, Protein: 17.5 g

---

FRENCH PEASANT BEETS SPIRALS

Servings: 2-4 | Cooking time: 30 minutes | Assembly time: 10 minutes

We tend to overlook beets as a healthy delicious winter vegetable. The mixture of red and golden beets is not only tasty, it's also quite visually stunning. These easy, quick to make, and appetizing beets and greens are simple to whip up, but come with a taste that seems like you've been working all day. The addition of beef broth to cook the shallots lightens the dish, but rounds out the taste. Feel free to add a little salt and pepper to taste, but be careful because the broth will make it quite salty.

Ingredients:

4-6 red and golden beets with greens, spiralized

1 bunch Swiss chard

3 Tbsp. beef broth

3 Tbsp. butter

1 shallot

2 Tbsp. sweet white wine

2 Tbsp. water

1 bunch parsley

Directions:

1. Clean the beets: Scrub and peel, then remove greens, chop coarsely, and set aside.

2. Spiralize the beets.

3. Remove the ribs from the Swiss chard, chop in bite sized pieces.

4. Toss with beet greens.

5. In a large frying pan heat broth and butter.

6. Sauté shallots until just translucent (about 5 minutes).

7. Add beet spirals to shallots.

8. Add salt and pepper to taste.

9. Reduce heat to low, and sauté beats for approximately 10-15 minutes, till they begin to glaze and become tender.

10. When beets are tender, add greens and chard.

11. Cook for 5 more minutes.

12. Add wine and cover, then cook until greens are wilting, adding water as necessary though the majority of the liquid should be absorbed into the greens.

13. When greens are wilted, and liquid absorbed, taste and adjust seasoning.

14. Ladle into large low bowls and garnish with parsley.

Nutritional Info: Calories: 93, Sodium: 126 mg, Dietary Fiber: 0.7, Total Fat: 8.8 g, Total Carbs: 1.9 g, Protein: 1.0 g

---

Lemon Chard Pasta

Servings: 2 | Prep Time: 10-15 minutes

This delicious lemony dish makes an excellent side to baked fish or pork. The slight tang of vinegar rounds out the flavor, holding up well against the slight bitterness of the chard.

Ingredients:

1 large zucchini, spiralized

1 bunch Swiss chard, chopped roughly

1/8 cup fresh cilantro, chopped

2 green onions, sliced thinly

1 Tbsp. lemon juice (or more, to taste)

1 Tsp. apple cider vinegar

1 Tsp. lemon zest

1/4 Tsp. paprika

1/4 Tsp. black pepper

Directions:

1. Spiralize the zucchini. Heat or cook as you prefer.

2. In a large skillet, sauté the chard in 1 Tbsp. water until limp, around 5 minutes. Remove from pan and set aside in a medium-sized serving bowl.

3. Combine the cilantro, vinegar, green onions, lemon zest, spices, and salt.

4.   Combine the pasta and the chard. Add the dressing and "toss" to coat.

Nutritional Info: Calories: 36, Sodium: 48 mg, Dietary Fiber: 3.0, Total Fat: 0.2 g, Total Carbs: 7.2 g, Protein: .7 g

---

Mediterranean Squash Stir-fry

Servings: 2 | Prep Time: 10 minutes

Stir-fries are one of the easiest, best tasting, and most wholesome dishes you can make in a short amount of time. This dish, filled with garlic and spices is visually stunning and delicious. For a slightly different take on the dish, try replacing the Italian seasoning with different spice blends like Greek seasoning.

Ingredients:

3 large zucchini, spiralized

2 large yellow squash, spiralized

1 large yellow onion

2 ripe tomatoes, diced or cut into rounds

2 large garlic cloves, minced

1 Tbsp. Italian seasoning

4 Tbsp. olive oil

Parmesan cheese

Directions:

1. Spiralize zucchini and squash.

2. Put 2 Tbsp. oil in a medium skillet.

3. Combine the "pasta" and main ingredients in the skillet. Cook on medium for 2-4 minutes until the vegetables are al dente.

4. Sprinkle with the Italian seasoning and cook another minute or so to blend the flavors.

5. If necessary, add another Tbsp. or two of oil.

6.   Sprinkle with Parmesan cheese and serve immediately at room temperature.

Nutritional Info: Calories: 402, Sodium: 51 mg, Dietary Fiber: 10.0, Total Fat: 30.5 g, Total Carbs: 29.9 g, Protein: 8.8 g

Mexican Slaw

Servings: 6 | Prep Time: 10 minutes

Crunchy, light, and a bit spicy, this slaw is a perfect accompaniment to fish tacos. If you like a bit more heat, you can add very finely diced jalapenos as an addition. Be careful though, because a big bite of jalapeno can be strong, even for those with a taste for very spicy things. For another variation, try roasting poblano chilies before dicing them. It makes the salad smoky and very rich.

Ingredients:

1/2 small head green cabbage, spiralized

1/2 small head Napa cabbage, spiralized

1 small bunch red radish

2 fresh poblano chilies (or hatch chiles)

Juice of 3 limes

1 bunch fresh cilantro, minced (about 2 cups)

1/4 Tsp. cayenne pepper

Directions:

1. Remove tough outer leaves from cabbages and spiralize.

2. Trim the radishes and slice thinly.

3. De-seed the peppers and cut into small dices.

4. Mix the cabbages, radishes, and peppers in a large bowl and set aside.

5.   Mix together the lime juice and pepper. Add the cilantro and let sit for 5 minutes. Pour vinaigrette over the vegetables then toss to blend. Either serve immediately, or chill for an hour.

Nutritional Info: Calories: 59, Sodium: 273 mg, Dietary Fiber: 2.0, Total Fat: 0.7 g, Total Carbs: 8.6 g, Protein: 4.3 g

---

PERFUMED NOODLES WITH FRUIT & NUTS

Servings: 4-6 | Prep Time: 10 minutes | Cooking Time: 12 minutes

An eastern-flavored dish, these noodles can easily be converted from a side dish to a main course with the addition of grilled lamb or chicken. Alternatively, pair with falafel or kebabs for a meal with international flare. The hint of coconut oil gives a bit of creaminess to the dish without overloading it with excess fat and the spices to provide depth and fragrance.

Ingredients:

4 cups squash, spiralized

2/3 cup dried chopped dried apricots

1/3 cup golden raisins

1/2 cup dried cherries (or cranberries)

1 Tbsp. coconut oil

1 Tsp. ground cardamom

1 thread saffron (if desired)

2/3 cup pistachio nuts, shelled and chopped

1/4 Tsp. ground pepper

Directions:

1. Spiralize the squash. (Thin strands recommended.)

2. Lightly sauté the chopped nuts in a Tbsp. of coconut oil.

3. Add the fruit and spices.

4. Add the squash noodles.

5. Sauté lightly until all the flavors blend.

6.   Serve immediately.

Nutritional Info: Calories: 300, Sodium: 481 mg, Dietary Fiber: 6.3, Total Fat: 16.4 g, Total Carbs: 38.9 g, Protein: 4.9 g

---

SOUTHWESTERN SPICED SWEET POTATO AND BEET SPIRALS WITH CHILLI-CILANTRO SOUR CREAM

Servings: 4 | Cooking time: 20 minutes | Assembly time: 10 minutes

Baked french fries style dishes are all the rage lately, but this dish really elevates the idea. The spices give the spirals a lovely, rich taste and baking them allows them to be both crispy and healthy. Be careful when cooking your spirals, they can burn very easily!

Ingredients:

Potato and Beet Spirals:

2 large sweet potatoes, spiralized

2 large beets, peeled and spiralized

1 large russet potato, spiralized

1 Tbsp. olive oil

2 Tsp. salt

1 1/2 Tsp. ground cumin

1 1/2 Tsp. chili powder

1 1/2 Tsp. paprika

1 1/2 Tsp. ground black pepper

1/2 -1 Tsp. cayenne to taste

Chili-Cilantro Sour Cream:

1 cup sour cream

2 Tbsp. lime juice

3 Tsp. sweet chili sauce

2 small garlic clove, minced or crushed

1 Tsp. salt

1 Tsp. black pepper

1 heaping Tbsp. cilantro

Directions:

Potato Spirals:

1. Preheat oven to 425° F.

2. Spiralize russet potato, sweet potatoes, and beets. (Thick strands recommended.).

3. Combine salt, cumin, chili powder, paprika, pepper, and cayenne.

4. Toss spices and cut potatoes and beets together till well coated.

5. Arrange all vegetables on a high-sided baking tray, in a single layer.

6. Bake on the middle rack of the oven until bottom is browned, about 8-10 minutes.

7. Turn potatoes and beets over and bake an additional 5-8 minutes.

8. Remove from oven and serve with chili-cilantro sour cream.

Chili-Cilantro Sour Cream:

1. Stir together all ingredients but cilantro, and mix very well.

2. Stir in cilantro.

Nutritional Info: Calories: 325, Sodium: 1,898 mg, Dietary Fiber: 5.5, Total Fat: 16.2 g, Total Carbs: 41.1 g, Protein: 5.1 g

SPICY SLAW

Servings: 6 | Prep Time: 15 minutes

A simple quick recipe, the pepper sauce in this dish really makes it stand out. Be sure to use a high quality sauce and experiment with what you like best. A vinegar-based pepper sauce will produce a totally different result than a sweet-chili based sauce. We recommend something on the more acidic side to work with the sweetness of the honey.

Ingredients:

4 cups green cabbage, spiralized

3 carrots, spiralized

3 Tbsp. apple cider vinegar

1 Tbsp. olive oil

1 Tsp. honey

1/2 Tsp. dry mustard

1/4 Tsp. pepper

1/2 Tsp. hot pepper sauce (or to taste)

Directions:

1. Spiralize the cabbage and carrots. Combine in a bowl.

2. Combine all the other ingredients with a whisk. Pour over the cabbage and carrots.

3. Refrigerate for at least an hour to blend flavors.

Nutritional Info: Calories: 53, Sodium: 36 mg, Dietary Fiber: 2.0 g, Total Fat: 2.5 g, Total Carbs: 7.8 g, Protein: 0.9 g

SESAME NOODLES

Servings: 8 | Prep Time: 20 minutes

By replacing large amounts of vegetable or olive oil with a much smaller amount of sesame oil, this recipe packs a punch of flavor without much grease. Try seasoned rice wine vinegar or adding a few Tbsp. of sake or mirin to the recipe for a slightly different taste. It also tastes great served chilled.

Ingredients:

4 cups zucchini or yellow squash, spiralized

1 bunch green onions, sliced thin

4 large garlic cloves, minced

3 Tbsp. honey

1/4 cup gluten-free soy sauce

1/3 cup rice vinegar

2 Tbsp. dark sesame oil

1 Tbsp. crushed red pepper

1 Tbsp. toasted sesame seeds

Directions:

1. Spiralize the zucchini or squash. (Thick strands recommended.)

2. Place the noodles in a large serving bowl.

3. Combine the sesame oil, vinegar, soy sauce, and honey in a small saucepan and bring to a boil. Add the crushed red pepper.

4. Pour hot mixture over the noodles. Toss to coat.

5. Garnish with sliced green onions and sesame seeds.

Nutritional Info: Calories: 81, Sodium: 31 mg, Dietary Fiber: 1.0, Total Fat: 4.2 g, Total Carbs: 9.7 g, Protein: 1.1 g

SQUASH SAUTÉ

Servings: 8 | Prep Time: 25-30 minutes

We find this recipe works best with the slightly sweet rich flesh of the summer squash as opposed to heartier winter squashes. The pairing of squash with onions and tomatoes makes it slightly Italian in taste without being overbearingly like pasta sauce. Still if you enjoy that, add a little more tomatoes and serve over zucchini noodles and you have a power-packed squash pasta!

Ingredients:

2 lbs. summer squash, spiralized

1 pound ripe Roma tomato, thinly sliced

1 medium yellow onion, thinly sliced

3 Tbsp. chicken broth

2 Tbsp. large garlic, minced

1/2 Tsp. crushed dried red pepper flakes

1 Tbsp. Italian seasoning

Parmesan cheese, for garnish

Directions:

1. Spiralize the squash (thick rings recommended).

2. Heat the broth in a large skillet. Sauté the onion and garlic until the onion is translucent.

3. Add the tomatoes and sauté until the tomatoes have released their juices.

4. Add the squash and sauté for another 1-2 minutes.

5. Stir in the Italian seasoning and the pepper flakes.

6. Serve hot.

Nutritional Info: Calories: 47, Sodium: 25 mg, Dietary Fiber: 2.2 g, Total Fat: 1.0 g, Total Carbs: 9.0 g, Protein: 2.0 g

---

ROASTED VEGETABLE SNACKS

Servings: 10 | Prep Time: 25 minutes

These crunchy little bits are healthy, delicious, and easy. Experiment with vegetables to find which ones you like best. We recommend turnips, beets, and sweet potatoes.

Ingredients:

---

1 large butternut squash, peeled and spiralized

1 Tbsp. olive oil

1 Tbsp. curry powder

1/2 Tsp. garlic powder

1 Tsp. chili powder

Directions:

---

1. Preheat oven to 450° F

2. Spiralize squash.

3. Combine the olive oil and spice in a large Ziplock bag.

4. Add the vegetable strands and shake well to coat evenly.

5. Arrange the strands on a baking sheet that has been brushed with olive oil or coated with cooking spray.

6. Roast until crispy.

7. Let cool then break up. The resulting crunchies will remind you of the crisp noodles that garnish Chinese chicken salad.

Nutritional Info: Calories: 22, Sodium: 4 mg, Dietary Fiber: 0.6, Total Fat: 1.5 g, Total Carbs: 2.2 g, Protein: 0.3 g

---

13

MAIN DISHES

"The table is a meeting place, a gathering ground, the source of sustenance and nourishment, festivity, safety, and satisfaction. A person cooking is a person giving: Even the simplest food is a gift."

Laurie Colwin

BAKED CHICKEN PARMESAN WITH NOODLES

Servings: 4 | Prep Time: 60 minutes

Traditionally, chicken Parmesan is fried in butter or oil, prior to being baked. This oven-only dish reduces the fat by removing the frying step. The panko breadcrumbs, as opposed to traditional breadcrumbs, add a bit of extra crunch, and baking till the chicken is golden brown makes that even more dramatic. It's not necessary to top with mozzarella cheese, but if you do try broiling for those last few minutes rather than baking!

Ingredients:

3 large zucchini, spiralized

3 boneless chicken breasts

2 eggs, beaten

1/2 cup dried Parmesan cheese

1/2 cup panko breadcrumbs

3 Tbsp. Italian seasoning

4-6 ounces tomato paste

8 oz tomato sauce

1/2 cup low-fat mozzarella cheese, grated if desired

Directions:

1. Preheat oven to 350° F.

2. Combine Parmesan cheese and panko breadcrumbs.

3. Cut chicken breasts in thirds. Dip them in the beaten egg, then into the cheese and breadcrumb mixture.

4. In a saucepan mix the tomato paste, Italian seasoning, and tomato sauce. Add salt and pepper to taste. Heat on medium heat till bubbling then reduce to low.

5. Arrange breaded chicken in a large glass-baking dish with 1/2 inch of space between pieces.

6. Bake about 25 minutes, until chicken is cooked through and golden brown.

7. Remove chicken from oven, top with the Mozzarella cheese.

8. Bake 5 additional minutes to melt and brown cheese.

9. Spiralize the zucchini. If softer noodles are desired, blanche for 1-2 minutes. Otherwise leave raw.

10. Serve the Parmesan chicken over the pasta and top with tomato sauce.

Nutritional Info: Calories: 302, Sodium: 547 mg, Dietary Fiber: 5.7 g, Total Fat: 10.7 g, Total Carbs: 25.6 g, Protein: 29.7 g

---

Baked Eggs with Spiralized Jicama

Servings: 6 | Prep time: 30 minutes | Cooking time: 30 minutes

A lacto-ovo vegetarian dish, it is perfect for people who love big flavors, without a lot of fat. The jicama is crunchy and fresh. The egg provides a hint of richness, to go with the acidity of the tomato broth. There are no added oils or cheese which add heaviness to so many dishes. This one is so tasty it doesn't need any of that!

Ingredients:

1 large jicama, spiralized

3 bell peppers red, green, and orange, thinly sliced

1 medium red onion, thinly sliced

2 beef steak tomatoes, cut into wedges

8 large garlic cloves, minced

1 jalapeño with seeds, halved lengthwise

1/4 cup fresh basil leaves

2 Tbsp. fresh oregano leaves

1 1/2 Tsp. chili powder

1 Tsp. paprika

6 large eggs

Salt and freshly ground black pepper to taste

Directions:

1. Start by adding bell peppers and onion to a large heavy bottomed pan. Cook stirring occasionally until they soften and just start to turn brown, about 10 minutes. If they stick, add 1-2 Tbsp. water to release.

2. Add tomato wedges, garlic, jalapeno, basil, oregano, chili powder, and paprika.

3.   Reduce heat to low, and cook stirring occasionally, until vegetables are softened, and the liquid in the pan have thickened some (about 25 minutes).

4.   Preheat oven to 400° F.

5.   Put bell pepper mixture in a 13 x 9 baking dish, spreading it out evenly.

6.   Make 6 evenly-spaced hollows in the mixture, large enough to hold an egg.

7.   Gently crack an egg into each one.

8.   Season with salt and pepper to taste.

9.   Put in the oven, then bake until egg whites are hardened and egg yolks are just starting to solidify. This will take about 15 minutes.

10. Remove from oven, and let sit 2-3 minutes to cool.

11. Spiralize the jicama. (Thick strands recommended.) Place into individual plates to make little nests of jicama strands.

12. Serve eggs over jicama nests.

13. Remember eggs will continue to cook as the dish sits out, so for softer eggs serve immediately.

Nutritional Info: Calories: 195, Sodium: 91 mg, Dietary Fiber: 13.1 g, Total Fat: 5.8 g, Total Carbs: 27.9 g, Protein: 9.5 g

---

BEEF PAPRIKASH WITH SQUASH NOODLES

Servings: 2 | Prep Time: 3 hours

This meaty rich dish relies on the flavor from the beef in it, so choose high quality lean cuts. When searing, let the cubes sit a little extra time on each side to develop a browned crust. Some crunchy bits will be left in the pan, so use water to deglaze the pan and scrape up all that goodness!

Ingredients:

4 yellow squash, spiralized

1/2 pounds stew beef, cut into cubes

2 cups beef broth

8 Roma tomatoes, seeded and diced

2 large yellow onions, diced

1 green bell pepper, seeded and diced

2 large garlic cloves, minced

3 Tbsp. paprika (or to taste)

2 Tsp. caraway seeds

Directions:

1. Preheat oven to 350° F.

2. Spiralize the squash into thick noodles.

3. Sear the beef cubes in the bottom of a Dutch oven, or a heavy oven-safe pan. Beef will stick slightly as it sears. Add 1-2 Tsp. water to release it, scrape up all browned bits. Push the beef cubes to the side then sauté the onions, bell pepper, and garlic cooking until the onions are translucent.

4. Add the tomatoes and beef stock.

5. Roast at 350° F for 2-2 1/2 hours until the beef is tender that it can be shredded with a fork.

6. Place the noodles into boiling water for a couple minutes, just enough to warm them.

7. Serve the paprikash over warmed "noodles."

Nutritional Info: Calories: 504, Sodium: 836 mg, Dietary Fiber: 15.2 g,

Total Fat: 14.2 g, Total Carbs: 60.3 g, Protein: 40.2 g

BEEF PHO

Servings: 4 | Prep Time: 25-30 minutes

Usually served with rice noodles, the substitution of squash noodles makes this recipe healthier, and higher in both fiber and nutrients. Remember, the longer you simmer the broth the better the flavor will be. If you prefer, you can slice the beef very thinly and pour the boiling broth over it, allowing it to cook almost instantly, but remain rare.

Ingredients:

2 cups yellow squash, spiralized

8 cups low sodium beef broth

4 cups water

3/4 pound flank steak, very thinly sliced

1 medium yellow onion, sliced

4-6 garlic cloves, minced

1 2-inch piece ginger root, grated

2 wholes cloves

1 cinnamon stick

2 Tbsp. fish sauce

For garnish: chopped green onions, thinly sliced jalapeno peppers, chopped cilantro, lime, wedges

Directions:

1. Spiralize the squash.

2. Combine broth, water, and spices in a large stockpot. Bring to a boil over high heat, then cover the pan and reduce the heat. Simmer for half an hour, stirring occasionally.

3.   Add the noodles and beef to the pot, return to a boil just long enough to cook the beef, about 1-2 minutes if the beef is sliced very thin. Remove the cinnamon stick, then serve hot with garnishes as desired.

Nutritional Info: Calories: 299, Sodium: 2,362 mg, Dietary Fiber: 1.9, Total Fat: 9.9 g, Total Carbs: 13.3 g, Protein: 36.0 g

---

CABBAGE AND APPLE SAUTÉ

Servings: 4 | Prep Time: 30 minutes

Replacing the more traditional pork bacon with turkey bacon lightens this recipe while still retaining its rich savory taste. Make sure to drain any fat off well to avoid adding extra fat to the dish. If the onions start to stick to pan, add a few Tsp. of water to release them.

Ingredients:

1 medium cabbage head, spiralized

2 tart apples

1/2 pound turkey bacon

1 large yellow onion, coarsely chopped

1 cup water

1-2 Tbsp. lemon juice

1 small bay leaf

Freshly ground pepper

Directions:

1. Fry bacon until crisp. Very little fat should render off.

2. If fat renders off, drain skillet well but do not wipe out, leaving a little liquid to cook onions in.

3. Spiralize the cabbage.

4. Place the chopped onion in the skillet.

5. Stirring frequently, cook onions until they are translucent being careful not to let them stick to the pan.

6. Add the cabbage and the bay leaf.

7. Cover and reduce heat.

8. Simmer for 20-30 minutes until the cabbage is tender but still a bit crisp.

9. While simmering the cabbage, spiralize the apples into strands. Squeeze 1-2 Tbsp.. of fresh lemon juice over the apple spirals and set aside.

10. When the cabbage is ready remove bay leaf and mix in the apple noodles.

11. Place the hot mixture in dish and garnish with bacon.

12. There's no need to add salt to this dish; the bacon fat will supply plenty of sodium.

Nutritional Info: Calories: 141, Sodium: 447 mg, Dietary Fiber: 4.4 g, Total Fat: 1.9 g, Total Carbs: 16.6 g, Protein: 11.6 g

---

Cabbage "Spaghetti" with Turkey Sauce

Servings: 4 | Prep Time: 30 minutes

Unlike traditional spaghetti, this cabbage pasta is light, fresh, and crispy, an excellent compliment to the rich tomato and turkey sauce.A twist on an old classic, this is sure to become a family favorite! Plus, it only takes a half hour to make.

Ingredients:

1 medium head cabbage, spiralized

3/4 cup cauliflower, spiralized

1 cup water

1 pound lean ground turkey

1 yellow onion, diced

2 garlic cloves, minced

1 medium can (15-ounces) diced tomato

3 Tbsp. low-sodium beef stock

2 Tbsp. apple cider vinegar

1 Tsp. thyme

2 Tsp. paprika

2 Tbsp. olive oil

Directions:

1. Spiralize the cabbage then sauté in a large skillet with the water until the cabbage is translucent.

2. Spiralize the cauliflower into "rice." Cook the cauliflower rice in boiling water for five minutes or until soft. Remove from heat and drain.

3. Fry the ground turkey till brown, then drain very well. Set aside. Drain excess oil out of pan, but do not wipe out leaving just enough oil to sauté onions in.

4. In the same pan, cook the onion and garlic until the onion is translucent.

5. Add the tomatoes, thyme, paprika, vinegar, and diced tomatoes.

6. Stir and continue cooking until the sauce thickens, about 10 minutes.

7. Stir in the ground turkey.

8. Add the cauliflower "rice" to the mixture and heat through.

9. Pour the meat mixture over the sautéed cabbage.

Nutritional Info: Calories: 278, Sodium: 283 mg, Dietary Fiber: 3.7, Total Fat: 15.4 g, Total Carbs: 10.7 g, Protein: 26.3 g

---

CHICKEN CURRY WITH CAULIFLOWER "RICE"

Servings: 4 | Prep Time: 30 minutes

A Thai-style curry dish, the addition of light coconut milk adds creaminess coupled with healthy fats. This dish is heavy on the spices, but don't be afraid to add a little more to your taste. We recommend trying a pinch of cayenne pepper, if you like heat. You can also try frying the cauliflower "rice" for a crispier texture.

Ingredients:

1 head cauliflower, spiralized

1 pound skinless chicken breasts or turkey cutlets

1 cup light coconut milk

1 large yellow onion, diced

2 garlic cloves, minced

2 Tsp. tomato paste (no sugar)

3 Tsp. curry powder

1 Tsp. cumin

1 Tsp. turmeric

1 Tsp. ginger

1/4 Tsp. cinnamon

2 Tbsp. olive oil

Directions:

1. Spiralize the cauliflower into "rice."

2. In a heavy pan or wok, sauté the onion and garlic in 1 Tbsp. of coconut milk until the onion is translucent.

3. Add all the spices and cook through. (The mixture will be a lovely golden color.)

4. Add the chicken and cook until completely cooked through.

5. Add the tomato paste and stir well.

6. Add the coconut milk and continue to cook (stirring frequently) until the chicken is completely cooked and the sauce has thickened.

7. Spoon the chicken and sauce over the Cauliflower rice.

Nutritional Info: Calories: 383, Sodium: 76 mg, Dietary Fiber: 4.7, Total Fat: 25.9 g, Total Carbs: 12.7 g, Protein: 28.8 g

CHICKEN VEGGIE ALFREDO

Servings: 4 | Prep Time: 20 minutes

Alfredo sauce is delicious, filling, and rich. Coupled with fresh vegetables, its also quite healthy and part of a perfect meal. This rich creamy sauce tops zucchini and chicken in an excellent compliment and makes either a great side dish or a main course in and of itself.

Ingredients:

3 zucchini, spiralized

2 chicken breasts, grilled on a barbecue or table top grill or baked, then cut into pieces

1 cup low-sodium chicken broth

1/2 cup whole milk

1/2 cup cream

3 Tbsp. olive oil

1 cup freshly grated Parmesan cheese (don't use dried parmesan)

4 garlic cloves, minced (or 2 Tsp. prepared minced garlic)

3 Tbsp. cornstarch (or substitute rice starch or all purpose flour)

Freshly ground black pepper

Directions:

1. Start with the chicken pieces at room temperature.

2. Spiralize zucchini.

3. Bring a pot of water to a boil.

4. Add olive oil to a pan and sauté the minced garlic for about a minute. Add the cornstarch and stir to combine. Cook for another two minutes, stirring occasionally over medium heat.

5. Pour the chicken broth into the garlic mixture slowly. Use a whisk to beat the mixture until its smooth. Add the milk and

cream then whisk until smooth and thickened. Simmer for another minute then add the cheese, stirring constantly until melted.

6. Add the fresh pepper and stir one more time. Turn off the heat.

7. Boil the vegetable pasta strands for 2-3 minutes. Drain and put into a large bowl.

8. Add the chicken pieces then pour the sauce over everything.

9. Toss to combine and serve immediately.

Nutritional Info: Calories: 306, Sodium: 334 mg, Dietary Fiber: 1.7, Total Fat: 20.9 g, Total Carbs: 13.7 g, Protein: 18.3 g

---

CHILI CINCINNATI STYLE

Servings: 8 | Prep Time: 20 minutes

Using half turkey sausage as opposed to all ground beef both lightens this dish and adds depth of flavor. Choose all-turkey sausage not one that has other meats mixed in. When cooking it, leave it a little longer than you'd expect to let it develop a crispy brown crust. This adds a rich taste without needing to add butter or oil.

Ingredients:

2 zucchini, spiralized

2 pounds lean ground beef

1 pound ground turkey sausage

4 pounds tomatoes, de-seeded and chopped

1 large yellow onion, chopped

1 green bell pepper, chopped

1 jalapeno pepper, diced

2-3 large garlic cloves, minced or crushed

4 Tbsp. chili powder

2 Tbsp. cumin

2 Tsp. paprika

1 Tsp. salt

1 Tsp. ground black pepper

Directions:

1. Spiralize the zucchini.

2. Brown the beef in a large frying pan and drain very well. Pat with a paper towel to remove excess fat and set aside.

3. In the same pan, brown the turkey. Drain well as above.

4. Put both meats into a large saucepan.

5. Add the chopped vegetables.

6. Add chili, cumin, paprika, salt and pepper.

7. Cover and cook for 4 – 6 hours over medium heat, stirring occasionally.

8. If the mixture gets too thick, add water, 1/2 cup at a time.

9. When ready to serve, toss the noodles into a pot of boiling water for 3-5 minutes (long enough to heat through without losing their al dente texture).

10. Ladle chili over warmed "noodles" to serve.

Nutritional Info: Calories: 353, Sodium: 669 mg, Dietary Fiber: 5.8 g, Total Fat: 12.2 g, Total Carbs: 17.1 g, Protein: 44.8 g

CURRIED CHICKEN WITH PASTA

Servings: 4 | Prep Time: 25-30 minutes

Yogurt is a delicious accompaniment for most meat, especially when cooked in curry. This recipe uses non-fat yogurt, which adds richness without a great deal of fat. For a more daring cook, try mixing your own curry blend! Spices can be found at local Asian or Middle Eastern markets, and you can put together the seasoning that fits your taste.

Ingredients:

6 large carrots, spiralized

4 boneless & skinless chicken breasts, cut into bite-sized pieces

1 16 oz. container non-fat plain yogurt

2 medium yellow onions, diced

2 Tbsp. large garlic, minced

2 Tbsp. curry powder

1 Tsp. cumin

1 Tsp. turmeric

1 Tsp. ginger

1/2 Tsp. cayenne pepper

1/2 Tsp. cinnamon

2 Tbsp. olive oil

Directions:

1. Spiralize the carrots. Heat or cook as you prefer.

2. Heat oil in a large skillet, then sauté the onions and garlic until translucent and fragrant.

3. Add the curry powder and other spices. Mix well until everything is golden yellow.

4. Add the chicken pieces to the spiced mixture and continue to cook until the chicken is white and cooked all the way through.

5. Turn the heat off. Wait five minutes and stir in the yogurt, mixing well. (Don't skip the waiting period or the yogurt will separate.)

6. Serve the chicken curry over the carrot pasta.

Nutritional Info: Calories: 360, Sodium: 220 mg, Dietary Fiber: 5.7, Total Fat: 14.2 g, Total Carbs: 30.6 g, Protein: 33.8 g

---

Drunken Clams with Sausage

Serves 4 | Prep time: 10 minutes | Cooking time: 20 minutes

Cream, wine, and clams. Cooking doesn't get any better. This recipe is the best of both worlds--delicious broth and hearty clams. When cooking the sausage, let it brown a little more than you think you should. The crunchy, almost-burnt bits really ramp up the tastes in the dish.

Ingredients:

1 large yellow squash, spiralized

3 large zucchini, spiralized

4 dozen littleneck clams, cleaned very well and scrubbed

2 hot turkey sausages, casing removed and meat chopped fine

1 medium yellow onion, sliced thinly

4 celery stalks, chopped finely

1/2 small bulb of fennel, sliced thinly

5 small garlic cloves, chopped finely

1 1/2 cups dry white wine

3/4 sweet white wine

1/2 cup half and half or cream

10 large fresh tarragon leaves

1/2 cup chicken broth

1 Tbsp. parsley, finely chopped

Salt and pepper to taste

Directions:

1. Spiralize the zucchini and squash.

2. Heat a large saucepan over medium heat.

3. Add the onions and cook until soft (about 4 minutes). If onions begin to stick, add a few Tsp. of the broth to release them

4. Add the garlic, celery, and fennel and cook for 4-5 minutes.

5. Add the sausage meat and cook until browned (about 5 minutes).

6. Add both wines and chicken broth. Bring to a boil.

7. Add the tarragon.

8. Add clams, cover with a lid, and cook, shaking the saucepan occasionally to stir until clams are open, about 6 minutes.

9. Spoon clams into serving dish.

10. Stir parsley and cream into broth.

11. Season with salt and pepper to taste.

Assemble the dish:

1. Place squash noodles into low-sided bowls or soup plates. Spoon clams on top. Top with broth and serve.

Nutritional Info: Calories: 383, Sodium: 538 mg, Dietary Fiber: 5.4, Total Fat: 10.5 g, Total Carbs: 28.4 g, Protein: 31.0 g

---

"Drunken Noodles" with Chicken

Servings: 4 | Prep Time: 20 minutes

A spicy, salty dish full of Asian flavor, drunken noodles are named not because they have alcohol in them, but in traditional Thai culture, they are considered the perfect food to have while drinking. Usually served with noodles, the yellow squash replaces them perfectly, without altering the core tastes of the dish. There is no soy sauce in this dish, leaving it gluten free without any effort!

Ingredients:

4 cups yellow squash, spiralized

2 chicken breasts, cooked and shredded 2 dried red chili, de-seeded and chopped finely (or to taste)

2 dried red lime leaves, sliced very thinly

2 shallots, thinly sliced

4 garlic cloves, minced

1 1-inch piece of ginger, grated

4 ripe cherry tomatoes, halved

1 cup bok choy

2 cups bean sprouts

3-5 basil leaves, chopped

1/2 cup fresh cilantro, chopped

2 Tbsp. lime juice

1 Tbsp. brown sugar

1 Tbsp. rice vinegar

1 Tbsp. "fish sauce"

1/2 Tsp. "yellow bean sauce" (available in asian markets, substitute, soy sauce, if necessary)

Directions:

1. Combine the lime juice, brown sugar, vinegar, and sauces to make the stir-fry sauce.

2. Spiralize the squash into thick strands.

3. In a wok, heat a few Tbsp. of vegetable oil and add the noodles and the rest of the ingredients except the tomatoes, bean sprouts and cilantro.

4. If you don't have any kaffir lime leaves (available at any Asian market), you can substitute a small bay leaf and about a Tbsp. of lime zest in a pinch.

5. Stir fry for two minutes, then add the tomatoes, bean sprouts, cilantro, and stir-fry sauce.

6. Stir-fry until everything is heated through.

7. If the dish seems too salty, add a little more lime juice. Garnish with additional cilantro.

Nutritional Info: Calories: 296, Sodium: 505 mg, Dietary Fiber: 5.0, Total Fat: 7.4 g, Total Carbs: 30.7 g, Protein: 31.0 g

---

ETHIOPIAN-INSPIRED SPICY CHICKEN STEW

Servings: 4 | Prep time: 20 minutes | Cooking time: 2 hours

Similar to doro wot, this stew substitutes skinless & boneless chicken breast for the more traditional & fattier, dark meat legs and thighs. There's no need for high-fat additions. However, there are so many varied spices, it gives this dish a complexity that makes it hard to believe how healthy it is. Ethiopian food gets better the longer you cook it, so try not to rush making this dish. Toasting the spices is particularly important so don't skip that step.

Ingredients:

3 large carrots, spiralized

1 large yellow squash, spiralized

1/4 Tsp. ground coriander

1/2 Tsp. ground fenugreek seeds

1/2 Tsp. black ground pepper

1/8 Tsp. ground allspice

1/8 Tsp. ground cardamom

1/8 Tsp. ground cloves

1/4-1/2 Tsp. ground cayenne pepper, to taste

1/4 Tsp. cinnamon

1/2 Tsp. ground turmeric

1 Tsp. fresh ginger, grated

1 medium yellow onion, grated or chopped finely

3 Tbsp. chicken broth

28 ounces can whole peeled tomatoes with juice

1 Tbsp. dry red wine

1 garlic clove, minced

3 skinless & boneless chicken breasts

4 hard boiled eggs

Salt to taste

Directions:

1. In a small bowl, mix all spices except salt.

2. Season the chicken breasts with salt and pepper then cut into strips.

3. In a deep frying pan, sauté chicken in chicken broth until browned all over.

4. Remove the chicken from the pan and lower the heat to medium, then add onions and ginger.

5. Cook for approximately 5 minutes, or till slightly translucent but not golden.

6. Add the dry spice mixture and cook for an additional 1-3 minutes until fragrant.

7. Add the tomatoes and juice. Chop down with a spatula.

8. Add the garlic and wine. Stir well.

9. Add the chicken back to the pan, then turn the heat down to low.

10. Simmer for 1 1/2 - 2 hours on low, uncovered, until sauce is thick.

11. Spiralize the carrots and squash. Heat or cook as preferred, then set aside.

12. 5 minutes before serving time, peel the eggs and add to the stew. It should be long enough to be fully heated through, and slightly colored from the sauce.

13. Serve on top of vegetable noodles.

Nutritional Info: Calories: 270, Sodium: 266 mg, Dietary Fiber: 6.3, Total Fat: 7.7 g, Total Carbs: 20.3 g, Protein: 28.0 g

Florentine Potato Pasta Casserole

Servings: 6 | Prep Time: 90 minutes

A wonderful cold-weather dish, this potato gratin is easy to make and tastes like you worked all day. Want a bit more of a kick? Add 1-2 Tsp. cayenne pepper to the broth and spinach mixture as you cook it.

Ingredients:

4 cups baking potatoes, spiralized

1 package sliced mushrooms (about 2 cups)

4 cups chicken broth

1 Tbsp. olive oil

1 medium yellow onion, chopped

1 large garlic clove, minced

1 10 package oz frozen chopped spinach, thawed, drained and squeezed dry

2 1/2 cups 1% milk

1/3 cup shredded low-fat sharp cheddar

1/2 Tsp. black pepper

Directions:

1. Preheat oven to 350° F.

2. Spiralize the potatoes.

3. Coat a baking dish (approx 11 x 7) with non-stick cooking spray.

4. In a large skillet heat the onions, mushrooms, and garlic in 1 Tbsp. broth until the onion is translucent and the onions have started to "shrivel."

5. Add the broth and black pepper. Continue to sauté over medium-high heat until the broth has been absorbed or evaporated.

6. Stir in the spinach.

7. Begin layering the potatoes into the prepared baking dish. Cover with a layer of the spinach/mushroom mixture.

8. Cover with 1/2 of the cheese mixture.

9. Add another layer of potatoes and the rest of the spinach mixture.

10. Combine the milk, eggs, and cornstarch.

11. Pour over the layers making sure everything is moist.

12. Bake in the pre-heated oven for 1 hour.

13. Top the casserole with the rest of the cheese and bake for another 15-20 minutes until the cheese is bubbling and golden brown.

14. Remove from oven and let sit for 5 minutes before serving.

Nutritional Info: Calories: 430, Sodium: 976 mg, Dietary Fiber: 15.1, Total Fat: 10.6 g, Total Carbs: 67.5 g, Protein: 26.2 g

---

Funky Low Fat Chicken With Sesame Noodles

Servings: 4 | Prep time: 3 hours (for marinade) | Cooking time: 30 minutes

An Asian flavored veggie pasta with deliciously marinated chicken. This recipe is quick, easy, and healthy. Sugar is replaced with honey, because it tastes sweeter and can be used with moderation. Sesame oil can be reduced to a bare minimum to give flavor without adding excess fat. It is not necessary to use any unless you want to, but since there are so many other spices, it won't even be missed.

Ingredients:

Noodles:

3 large zucchini, spiralized

1/2 cup gluten free soy sauce

2 Tbsp. sesame oil (if desired)

3 Tbsp. honey

3 scallions, thinly sliced

1/4 cup or more sesame seeds

Chicken:

1/4 cup gluten free soy sauce

1/4 cup gluten free teriyaki sauce

2 garlic cloves, minced

2 Tbsp. honey

1 Tsp. fresh ginger, chopped

4 boneless & skinless chicken breasts

2-3 Tbsp. sesame oil (if desired)

Directions:

Zucchini Pasta:

1. Spiralize zucchini.

2. Heat a pot of lightly salted water to boiling. Add zucchini noodles and blanch for 3-4 minutes until just tender.

3.   Rinse well and set aside.

4.   In a small bowl mix sesame oil, honey, and soy sauce. Whisk until the honey has totally incorporated.

5.   Pour this over noodles and toss well.

6.   Add scallions and sesame seeds. Toss again.

7.   Set aside for flavors to mix while preparing chicken.

Chicken:

1.   In a medium bowl mix soy sauce, teriyaki sauce, garlic, brown sugar, and ginger.

2.   Whisk until sugar is totally dissolved.

3.   Add chicken mixing well to coat.

4.   Cover and put in refrigerator for at least 2 hours to absorb flavor.

5.   When marinating is done, remove chicken from refrigerator.

6.   Heat a large frying pan with sesame oil over medium-high heat.

7.   Add the chicken in batches, so as not to crowd it and cook approximately 5 minutes on each side till cooked through. Add oil as needed.

8.   Set aside for 10 minutes to rest.

9.   Cut chicken into thin strips and serve on a bed of seasoned noodles.

Nutritional Info: Calories: 515, Sodium: 334 mg, Dietary Fiber: 3.1 g, Total Fat: 24.5 g, Total Carbs: 31.8 g, Protein: 44.1 g

GREEK LAMB PASTA

Servings: 6 | Prep Time: 50-60 minutes

This dish uses lamb as an alternative to more traditional ground beef and mixes in Greek flavors such as olives and Greek seasoning. To add a bit more flare, sprinkle crumbled low-fat feta cheese over the top before serving or substitute kalamata olives for black olives. You can also leave out the ground lamb and use the pasta as an accompaniment to lamb chops.

Ingredients:

4 cups zucchini or yellow squash, spiralized

1 pound ground lamb

1 can (4 oz) sliced black olives, drained

1 can (28 oz) can diced tomato

1 small can tomato paste

2 Tbsp. oregano (or Greek seasonings, blend)

3 large garlic cloves minced

1 large yellow onion, diced

1 large bell pepper, diced

Juice of one lemon

3 Tbsp. balsamic vinegar

Directions:

1. In a large saucepan brown the ground lamb. Drain well, but do not wipe out pan. Add the onion, bell pepper, garlic, and olives then cook until the onions become translucent.

2. Add the diced tomatoes, lemon juice, vinegar, and spices.

3. Simmer for 10 minutes, then stir in tomato paste.

4. Simmer another 10-20 minutes, adding small amounts of water if the sauce becomes too thick.

5.   Spiralize the zucchini or yellow squash. Heat or cook as desired.

6.   Serve over pasta and enjoy!

Nutritional Info: Calories: 201, Sodium: 282 mg, Dietary Fiber: 3.8 g, Total Fat: 6.0 g, Total Carbs: 13.5 g, Protein: 24.0 g

---

PASTA & TURKEY/CHIA SEED MEATBALLS

Servings: 4 | Prep Time: 50 minutes

Chia seeds are one of nature's super foods. Packed with good fats, vitamins, and dietary fiber. It adds punch to anything you're eating. These meatballs have a rich slightly nutty flavor that works well with the marinara sauce. There are no oils or fats added to this recipe, all of which are derived from the meat, so pick lean options to keep waistline friendly.

Ingredients:

Pasta:

1 large zucchini, spiralized

Meatballs:

1 pound lean ground turkey (can use Italian seasoned if desired)

4 Tbsp. tomato paste

2 Tbsp. chia seeds

3 garlic cloves, minced

2 Tsp. oregano

2 Tsp. basil

1 Tsp. black pepper

Marinara:

1 medium yellow onion, diced

1 garlic clove, (crushed)

1 sprig fresh rosemary, (chopped)

1/4 cup lemon juice

1/2 cup chicken stock

1 can (12 oz) tomato, diced

1 can (12 oz) tomato sauce

1/2 Tsp. salt

1/2 Tsp. black pepper

Directions:

1. Spiralize zucchini.

Prepare Chia Meatballs:

1. Mix all the ingredients. Let sit for 10 minutes.

2. Heat a large skillet to low-medium.

3. Shape the meat mixture into small balls (about eight) and brown in skillet, turning each meatball at least 3 times so they brown evenly. Remove the meatballs from heat, still slightly rare. Set aside.

4. Drain skillet of any fat, but do not rinse out.

Prepare the Marinara:

1. In the same skillet, sauté the onion until it's translucent. If it starts to stick, add 1-2 Tsp. water to release.

2. Add the rosemary and garlic then cook for another 2-4 minutes.

3. Add the lemon juice and chicken stock, then the diced tomatoes, tomato sauce, salt & pepper. Mix well.

4. Simmer over medium heat until sauce begins to thicken (about 20 minutes).

5. Reduce heat to low and add meatballs to the pan. Cook for 10 minutes or until meatballs are cooked thoroughly.

6. Divide pasta and sauce between two plates and top with meatballs and sauce.

Nutritional Info: Calories: 265, Sodium: 842 mg, Dietary Fiber: 7.1 g, Total Fat: 11.0 g, Total Carbs: 15.2 g, Protein: 27.4 g

---

PASTA CAJUN STYLE

Servings: 4 | Prep Time: 25-30 minutes

A simple off-the-cuff version of jambalaya. This dish mixes up rapidly and tastes great. Like traditional jambalaya, the meat can be substituted with anything available like white fish, scallops, different kinds of sausage, chicken, and pork can be used instead of the shrimp and Andouille, as long as you keep the spice blend the same.

Ingredients:

4 large zucchinis, spiralized

1/2 cup plus 3 Tbsp. chicken broth

2 - 2 Andouille-style sausages, cooked and cut into 1/2 inch pieces

8 ounces raw shrimp, deveined

1/2 red bell pepper, chopped

1/2 green bell pepper, chopped

2 garlic cloves, crushed

1/2 yellow onion, diced

3 Tbsp. cajun spice, mixes

Directions:

1. Spiralize zucchini. Heat or cook as you prefer.

2. In a large skillet, heat the 3 Tbsp. broth over medium heat.

3. Sauté the onions and peppers with 1 Tbsp. of Cajun spice mix. When the vegetables are tender and the onions is translucent, set aside in a bowl.

4. Add the shrimp and another Tbsp. of the spice mix to the same pan and sauté until the shrimps are cooked through. Add the cooked shrimps to the sautéed vegetables in the bowl.

5. Add the sausage pieces to the skillet, along with the last Tbsp. of Cajun spice. Sauté until the sausages are cooked thoroughly. Add the sausages to the bowl of ingredients on the side.

6. Add prior cooked ingredients and chicken broth. Adjust amount of chicken broth to desired consistency.

7. Serve sauce over the pasta.

Nutritional Info: Calories: 346, Sodium: 1,246 mg, Dietary Fiber: 4.2 g,

Total Fat: 14.7 g, Total Carbs: 14.7 g, Protein: 29.6 g

PASTA E FAGILO

Servings: 8 | Prep Time: 45 minutes

One generally doesn't think of canned beans as the staple of a healthy diet. It's been shown that if using low-sodium well-rinsed beans, it is actually remarkably good for you. This soup mixes the high protein qualities of beans with the rich, Italian flavors of turkey sausage and tomatoes. By using turkey sausage and draining it well, you are cutting out the highest fat element. By rinsing the beans, you're reducing the salt without diminishing flavor.

Ingredients:

1 cup zucchini or yellow squash, spiralized

1 pound spicy Italian sausage, turkey or pork (if using links, remove casing)

4 cups chicken broth

1 cup water

4 carrots, sliced into coins

1 large yellow onion, diced

4 garlic cloves, crushed

1 can (16 oz) tomato sauce

1 can (15 oz) tomato, diced

1 can (15 oz) kidney beans

1 can (15 oz) cannellini or navy beans

1 Tbsp. Italian seasoning

Directions:

1. Spiralize zucchini or squash.

2. Crumble the sausage into the bottom of a large stockpot or Dutch oven then brown over medium heat. Drain off the excess fat. Add garlic, onions, and carrots. Cook until the vegetables are tender (about 4 minutes). Stir occasionally.

3. Add the water, chicken stock, tomato sauce, and diced tomatoes (including juice). Stir in the Italian seasoning and bring to a boil.

4. Drain and rinse the canned beans, then add to the soup. Add the beans to the pot and reduce heat. Simmer for 2-3 minutes, then toss in the noodles and simmer another 1-2 minutes. Serve hot.

Nutritional Info: Calories: 141, Sodium: 495 mg, Dietary Fiber: 1.8 g, Total Fat: 3.2 g, Total Carbs: 8.4 g, Protein: 18.8 g

---

PASTA PUTTANESCA

Servings: 4 | Prep Time: 20 minutes

The slightly inappropriate name of this pasta comes from the story that its inventor, an Italian chef, was beset by hungry customers right as he was about to close. They told him to make "anything" and he created this tangy, salty, savory dish out of what he had left in the kitchen. If you like your food salty, you can also add capers to the sauce, when you add the olives.

Ingredients:

4 cups zucchini or yellow squash, spiralized

6 anchovies canned in oil (half a 2-oz. can)

28 ounces (1 can), crushed tomatoes

1/2 cup pitted black olives, chopped

2 Tbsp. tomato paste

4 garlic cloves, minced

1 Tsp. crushed red pepper flakes (or more to taste)

1 Tbsp. Italian seasoning

1/2 small yellow onion, minced

Directions

1. Drain the anchovies, reserving 2 Tsp. of oil.

2. Heat the olive oil in a large saucepan over medium-high heat and sauté the onions until they're soft and translucent, about 4-5 minutes. Add the garlic and the anchovies.

3. Stir and continue to cook. (The anchovies will literally "melt" into the oil.)

4. Add the can of crushed tomatoes (juice and all) along with the tomato paste, Italian seasoning, pepper flakes, and olives.

5.   Reduce heat and simmer for 20 minutes.

6.   Spiralize zucchini or squash. (Thin strands recommended.) If soft noodles are desired, blanche the squash for 1-2 minutes. Otherwise leave raw.

7.   Pour over pasta and serve immediately.

Nutritional Info: Calories: 435, Sodium: 8,887 mg, Dietary Fiber: 4.7, Total Fat: 24.6 g, Total Carbs: 15.7 g, Protein: 41.4 g

---

PASTA WITH ANCHOVY SAUCE

Servings: 6 | Prep Time: 10-15 minutes

While anchovies are high in fat, they're packed with the good kind-- Omega-3 fatty acids. Like avocados, this is one of the sources of fat you want to keep in your diet. This recipe is a little heavier than some, but it packs a punch of nutrients and flavor. Instead of oil as a carrier for the fish, we've used vegetable stock, to remove the less-beneficial fats.

Ingredients:

4 cups zucchini or yellow squash, spiralized

12 anchovy fillets, packed in olive oil (2-ounce can)

1/4 cup vegetable broth

1/4 cup olive oil

1 Tbsp. oil from anchovies

1 Tbsp. crushed red pepper flakes

Juice of one lemon

1/4 cup Italian parsley, minced

Directions:

1. Spiralize zucchini or squash.

2. Drain oil, reserving 1 Tbsp., and mince anchovies.

3. In a small saucepan, heat the minced anchovies in vegetable broth and reserved oil. Stir until the fish "melt" (about 5 minutes).

4. Stir in the pepper flakes and the rest of the olive oil.

5. Add the lemon juice and stir.

6.   Pour the hot sauce over the raw noodles and mix together.

Nutritional Info: Calories: 106, Sodium: 454 mg, Dietary Fiber: 0.9, Total Fat: 9.5 g, Total Carbs: 2.8 g, Protein: 4.0 g

---

Pasta with Charred Tomato Sauce

Servings: 2 | Prep Time: 75 minutes

Roasted garlic has a delicious, hearty, and rich flavor that can be achieved without the addition of oils or butters. A little water softens the cloves of the garlic and allows them to be removed from their papers with limited effort. The eggplant in this recipe makes the sauce meatier with the roasted garlic contributing to the "charred" name.

Ingredients:

1 large zucchini, spiralized

1/4 large eggplant, diced

2 Roma tomatoes, seeded and diced

4 large garlic cloves, peeled

1 1/2 Tbsp. olive oil

1/4 yellow onion, diced

5 basil leaves, chopped

Directions:

1. Preheat oven to 325° F.

2. Wrap 5 peeled garlic cloves in aluminum foil, along with 1/2 Tbsp. olive oil and a pinch of salt.

3. Bake garlic for 40-50 minutes, until browned and soft.

4. Sauté the diced eggplant until soft (10-12 minutes) in a large skillet. Set cooked eggplant aside.

5. Using the same pan, combine 2 of the roasted garlic cloves, the diced tomatoes, and the diced onion. Cook for 2-4 minutes, adding more olive oil if necessary.

6. Remove from heat and blend into a smooth paste in a food processor.

7. Spiralize the zucchini.

8. Combine the tomato mixture, the remaining garlic, and the pasta and cook over medium heat for another 2-4 minutes.

9. Garnish with the chopped basil.

Nutritional Info: Calories: 165, Sodium: 12 mg, Dietary Fiber: 3.7 g, Total Fat: 11.6 g, Total Carbs: 15.2 g, Protein: 4.0 g

---

PASTA WITH CLAMS

Servings: 2 | Prep Time: 45-50 minutes

This spicy delicious fresh clam dish is easy to make and easy to love. Cooking the clams in white wine gives them a fragrant, rich taste, and adding tomatoes makes the dish reminiscent of spicy Italian pastas. If you like a bit more kick, add red pepper flakes to the sauce.

Ingredients:

2 large zucchini, spiralized

1 large carrot

1/2 pound littleneck clams

2 Tbsp. fish or clam broth

1 12 oz. jar of spicy tomato sauce

1/4 cup dry white wine

1 garlic clove, minced

1 Tbsp. basil, chopped

Directions:

1. Spiralize the zucchini. Heat or cook, as you prefer.

2. Inspect clams and discard any with chipped or wide-open shells. If shells are partially open, tap on the shells to see if they close. If they do not, discard the clams.

3. Place clams in a large bowl and cover with cold water. Let soak for 25 minutes. Pull the clams one by one from the now-dirty water and rinse individually while scrubbing the shells to remove any remaining debris or sand. Repeat until all the clams are cleaned.

4. Refrigerate clams.

5. Add broth to a large saucepan and cook the garlic and onions until they are soft but not brown, about 1 minute.

6. Add the white wine and bring to a boil.

7. Add the cleaned clams (in their shells), cover and cook for 5-8 minutes until the shells have opened. Don't overcook; if a shell hasn't opened after 8 minutes, it's not going to, so discard it.

8. Remove the clams and set aside.

9. Strain the wine/clam broth and combine it with the tomato sauce in a medium saucepan. Bring to a boil.

10. Reduce heat, add the basil and simmer for another 5 minutes.

11. Combine the sauce and the clams and serve over the "pasta."

Nutritional Info: Calories: 572, Sodium: 2,927 mg, Dietary Fiber: 17.3 g,

Total Fat: 16.2 g, Total Carbs: 82.6 g, Protein: 17.7 g

Pesto Zucchini Pasta with Sausage

Servings: 3 | Prep Time: 15 minutes

Traditional pesto uses pine nuts, but this pesto has substituted walnuts to provide a unique flavor. Using the wine to deglaze the pan also adds dimension. You can also add additional basil, if you want a bit of a richer pesto sauce.

Ingredients:

3 zucchini, spiralized

1 (27-ounces) package hot Italian turkey sausage

1 cup fresh basil

1/2-3/4 cup walnuts

4 large garlic cloves, minced

3 Tbsp. dry white wine

Dash of salt

Directions:

1. Chop the sausages into bite-size pieces then brown and sear on all sides in a non-stick pan. Set aside.

2. Use 2 Tbsp. of white wine to deglaze sausage pan, scraping up all crispy bits.

3. Combine all the other ingredients and deglazed pan drippings in the bowl of a food processor. Blend until smooth.

4. Spiralize zucchini.

5. Warm the zucchini pasta in boiling water then drain and put in a large bowl.

6.   Toss with the pesto sauce and cooked pieces of sausage.

Nutritional Info: Calories: 1,045, Sodium: 1,983 mg, Dietary Fiber: 3.8 g,
Total Fat: 85.1g, Total Carbs: 10.6 g, Protein: 57.5 g

Pizza Pasta

Servings: 2 | Prep Time: 35-40 minutes

A quick and easy dish, this is guaranteed to please the most picky eaters. Even those who don't really like zucchini can eat this, because the noodles is hidden so well in the pizza sauce. Plus using homemade sauce reduces the excess sugars and additives that generally are in canned goods.

Ingredients:

2 zucchini, spiralized

2 large carrots

2 Italian chicken turkey sausages

14 ounces can tomato sauce

2 Tbsp. white vinegar

5 Tbsp. Italian seasoning

1 cup large yellow onion, diced

1 cup sliced mushrooms

1 bell pepper, diced

1/4 cup sliced black olives

4 garlic cloves, minced

Directions:

1. Spiralize zucchini. Heat or cook as you prefer.

2. Cut the sausages into 1-inch pieces and sauté in a medium skillet. Set aside.

3. In the same skillet, cook the onions until they are translucent, then add the diced pepper and sliced mushrooms.

4. Cook for another 5 minutes.

5. Add the tomato sauce, Italian seasoning, and vinegar.

6.   Mix in the cooked sausage pieces.

7.   Pour over the "pasta" and garnish with sliced olives.

Nutritional Info: Calories: 453, Sodium: 1,766 mg, Dietary Fiber: 10.9 g,

Total Fat: 21.8 g, Total Carbs: 41.9 g, Protein: 25.2 g

PORCINI AND ROSEMARY CRUSTED BEEF TENDERLOIN WITH PORT WINE SAUCE AND POTATO LINGUINI

Servings: 6-8 | Cooking time: 1 hour | Assembly time: 20 minutes

So many crusted beef recipes involve breadings or gluten-filled crusts, this alternative is delicious and delightful. Using dried mushrooms for the crust, it creates a beautiful, crispy outer layer without breadcrumbs or other agglutinated ingredients. The sauce is rich, and it is also makes a good accompaniment for the potato linguine.

Ingredients:

Tenderloin:

3 pounds beef tenderloin

1 ounce dried porcini mushrooms

2 Tbsp. fresh rosemary leaves, chopped finely

1 Tsp. black peppercorns

Salt to taste

Sauce:

1/2 ounce dried porcini mushrooms

3/4 cup water

1 medium shallot, chopped finely

1 cup port wine

1 cup heavy bodied red wine

2 rosemary springs

Salt to taste

Potato Linguini:

5-6 large russet potatoes,
spiralized

Salt to taste

Directions:

Tenderloin:

1. Salt tenderloin well, all over.

2. Refrigerate covered, for at least 4 hours but not more than 24 hours.

3. 30 minutes before roasting, remove from refrigerator to allow to come up to room temperature

4. Preheat oven to 400° F.

5. Combine mushrooms, rosemary, and peppercorns in a spice grinder or food processor (make sure mushrooms are totally dry so they pulverize well.)

6. Grind to a coarse powder.

7. Rub beef with mushroom rosemary powder.

8. Heat 1 Tbsp. oil in a heavy bottomed skillet.

9. Sear all sides of beef till brown and slightly crispy.

10. Transfer to a roasting pan.

11. Roast until meat thermometer in the thickest part reads 125° F (about 30 minutes).

12. Remove from oven and transfer to a cutting board.

13. Tent with foil and let rest for 15 minutes.

Sauce:

1. Reconstitute the mushrooms by placing the mushrooms in water for about 20 minutes, till swelled.

2. Strain liquid through a paper towel or coffee filter into a small bowl, reserving liquid.

3. Coarsely chop mushrooms.

4. In the skillet used for browning the meat, add shallots and chopped mushrooms.

5. Sauté over medium heat until shallots are soft and translucent 2-5 minutes.

6. Add port wine to deglaze the pan, scraping up all browned bits.

7. Add red wine, mushroom liquid, and rosemary.

8. Bring to a boil and cook on high heat uncovered, until sauce has reduced by about half to roughly 1 1/2 cups.

9. Add salt to taste.

10. Strain through a fine-meshed sieve, pushing on all solids to drain liquid.

11. Discard solids and put sauce back in a small sauce pan over medium heat

12. Set aside.

Potato Linguini:

1. Spiralize potatoes, skin on.

2. Boil a large pot of lightly salted water, and add potatoes.

3. Boil till tender, but not falling apart about 5-8 minutes.

4. Drain very well.

5. Reheat pan used to brown the meat and make the sauce base over medium heat.

6. Add potatoes to pan and sauté lightly till slightly crispy.

Assemble the Dish:

1. Cut rested tenderloin diagonal to the grain, in 1/4 inch slices.

2. Make a nest of potato linguini on the plate, top with sliced tenderloin.

3. Dress with port wine sauce.

4. Serve warm.

Nutritional Info: Calories: 628, Sodium: 250 mg, Dietary Fiber: 8.4, Total Fat: 16.2 g, Total Carbs: 50.8 g, Protein: 55.7 g

Quick and Easy Pasta Arrabiata

Servings: 4 | Prep Time: 60 minutes

With just a bit of heat, this rich pasta sauce pairs well with almost anything, but tastes best served over al dente zucchini noodles. Without the weight of traditional pasta, this dish is healthy, fresh, and vegetarian. Add more or less red pepper flakes depending on how spicy you want it to be. Remember, the longer you cook the sauce, the better the flavors will meld.

Ingredients:

4 cups zucchini, spiralized

Large (56 oz) can tomatoes (don't drain)

4 large garlic cloves, minced

1 bunch fresh basil, chopped (1/3-1/2 cup)

2 Tsp. crushed red pepper flakes (or more, to taste)

2 Tsp. water

Directions:

1. Spiralize the zucchini.

2. Combine all the ingredients except the basil and "pasta" in a large saucepan.

3. Simmer for half-hour to 45 minutes.

4. Add the basil and simmer for another 10 minutes.

5. While the sauce is on its final simmer, warm the pasta by cooking it for 2-3 minutes in a pot of boiling water.

6. Serve immediately. Garnish with Parmesan cheese and more pepper flakes if desired.

Nutritional Info: Calories: 122, Sodium: 30 mg, Dietary Fiber: 8.9, Total Fat: 0.8 g, Total Carbs: 25.5 g, Protein: 7.8 g

---

QUICK AND EASY PASTA WITH LEMON & RICOTT

Servings: 2 | Prep Time: 20 minutes

This recipe takes less time to make than it does to eat. The sauce is so tasty that a little bit goes a long way. The slightly sour lemony flavor, mixed with the richness of the ricotta makes the dish taste like it took hours, instead of minutes.

Ingredients:

4 cups zucchini or yellow squash, spiralized

2 quarts water

8 ounces container low-fat ricotta cheese

2 Tbsp. chicken broth

1/2 cup flat-leaf parsley, chopped

1/2 Tsp. black pepper

3 Tbsp. lemon juice

Zest of one lemon

Directions:

1.   Spiralize the zucchini or squash.

2.   Bring the water to boil in a large saucepan.

3.   Boil the pasta for 1-2 minutes until tender. Remove 1 cup of water from the pasta pot.

4.   Combine the cheese, broth and reserved pasta water, whisking until creamy.

5.   Drain the pasta and put in a large serving bowl.

6.   Add the parsley, pepper, lemon zest, lemon juice, and the cheese mixture.

7. Toss with tongs to mix.

8. Serve immediately.

Nutritional Info: Calories: 207, Sodium: 254 mg, Dietary Fiber: 3.2 g, Total Fat: 9.8 g, Total Carbs: 15.2 g, Protein: 16.6 g

---

ROSEMARY PORK RAGOUT WITH SWEET POTATO PASTA

Servings: 4 | Prep Time: 3.5 Hours

The important note with this dish is to buy high-quality lean pork. The leaner the meat, the better flavor you'll get and the healthier it will be. Searing the meat allows its natural juices to mix with the onion, removing the need for extra oils. A great cold-weather dish, it requires no additional fats to be added, and draws all its richness directly from the meat itself.

Ingredients:

6 sweet potatoes, peeled & spiralized

1 large yellow onion, roughly chopped

2 pounds lean pork roast, fat trimmed well

3 sprigs fresh rosemary, chopped (or 3 Tsp. dried rosemary)

2 large garlic cloves, minced

1 ounce can crushed tomato (no salt)

Dash of freshly ground black pepper

Directions:

1. Using a dry skillet, sear the pork on all sides. Leave long enough on each side that pork releases easily.

2. Remove the meat from the pan and set aside.

3. Combine the garlic, onion, and chopped rosemary and sauté in the same pan until the onion is translucent. Pork should have released just enough juice to easily sauté onions but if it doesn't, add 1-2 Tsp. water.

4. Combine the rosemary mixture with the meat in a large saucepan.

5. Pour in the crushed tomatoes juice and all.

6. Add the seared pork loin.

7. Bring the liquid to a boil, then cover and reduce heat.

8. Simmer until the pork begins to fall apart (about 3 hours).

9. Remove the cooked meat from the liquid and let cool slightly.

10. Shred the meat and return to the pot, simmering another five minutes until everything has warmed up again.

11. Spiralize the sweet potatoes.

12. Prepare or cook according to your preference. (Don't overcook or they'll get mushy).

13. Pour the Ragout over the pasta and garnish with additional rosemary sprigs if desired.

Nutritional Info: Calories: 437, Sodium: 572 mg, Dietary Fiber: 13.5 g,

Total Fat: 5.4 g, Total Carbs: 78.5 g, Protein: 19.1 g

Secret Ingredient Beef Stew

Servings: 8-10 | Cooking time: 3 hours | Assembly time: 20 minutes

Anchovies are a heavy hitter in terms of flavor and nutritional benefits. Packed with good fats and fatty acids. It is also rich, tasty, and adds dimension to this beef stew. Like all beef stews, it does better the longer it is cooked and more effectively if you sear the beef.

Ingredients:

5 - 5 1/2 pounds stew beef, cut into 2-3 inch pieces

2 leeks, washed and sliced thinly

1 large onion, diced

8 garlic cloves, minced or crushed

2 carrots, diced finely

4 celery stalks, diced finely

4 ounces white mushrooms, roughly chopped

1/4 cup tomato paste

2 anchovies

1/2 cup red wine vinegar

1 cup red wine

3 cups beef broth

1 cup canned whole tomatoes with juice

1 1/2 Tsp. salt

3 bay leaves

3/4 Tsp. dried thyme

1/3 cup chopped fresh parsley

1 large zucchini, spiralized

1 large yellow squash, spiralized

Salt and pepper to taste

Directions:

1. Season the beef with salt and pepper lightly.

2. Brown the beef over high heat, making sure to sear all sides well.

3. Remove and set aside. Drain pan very well, but do not rinse or wipe out.

4. Lower the heat and add all vegetables except zucchini.

5. Cook for 5-10 minutes until softened.

6. Stir in tomato paste and anchovies, then cook about 5 minutes to melt the tomato paste and anchovies, mixing it well.

7. Add the beef back to the pan and any juices that have drained.

8. Add the wine, vinegar, and tomatoes with juice.

9. Use a spatula or slotted spoon to break up the tomatoes.

10. Bring to a boil.

11. Add the stock, enough to cover the vegetables and beef in the pot (this may require slightly more than 3 cups).

12. Add salt, bay leaves, and thyme. Bring to a boil.

13. Simmer partially covered, about 2-3 hours.

14. Remove from heat and cool to room temperature, then put in the refrigerator.

15. When fully cold and fat has rendered to the top, skim off as much fat as possible.

16. Put back on low heat and reheat slowly.

17. Cook 20-30 minutes on low heat, just simmering.

18. Spiralize both zucchini and squash. Toss into stew and turn off heat.

19. Mix in half the parsley, then garnish with the remainder and serve.

Nutritional Info: Calories: 308, Sodium: 1,750 mg, Dietary Fiber: 5.9, Total Fat: 13.3 g, Total Carbs: 27.7 g, Protein: 16.3 g

---

SLOW COOKER ZUCCHINI PASTA WITH EGGPLANT SAUCE

Servings: 2 | Prep Time: 15 minutes

A play on eggplant parmigiana, this dish is wonderful to cook all day. Just fill your slow cooker in the morning and by dinner time, you've got a delicious and developed pasta sauce. If you're not fond of zucchini pasta, you can also serve this over spaghetti squash, for a slightly different taste.

Ingredients:

4 cups zucchini, spiralized

4 small ("baby") eggplants or one large one

1 medium yellow onion, chopped

1 can (28 oz) can Italian-style plum, tomato

3 large garlic cloves, chopped

1 4 can oz sliced mushrooms, drained

1/3 cup dry, red wine

1/3 cup water

1 1/2 Tsp. Italian seasoning

Directions:

1. Peel eggplant and dice into 1-inch cubes.

2. Combine all the ingredients, except the pasta and olives in a 5 1/2 quart slow cooker.

3. Cook on low-heat setting for 8 hours.

4. Spiralize the zucchini. If a softer noodle is desired, then blanche for 1-2 minutes, otherwise leave raw.

5.   Stir the olives into the sauce and pour over pasta.

Nutritional Info: Calories: 171, Sodium: 170 mg, Dietary Fiber: 10.8, Total Fat: 1.9 g, Total Carbs: 29.8 g, Protein: 6.8 g

---

Smoked Salmon Pasta with Lemon & Dill

Servings: 2 | Prep Time: 25 minutes

So many seafood pastas are full of heavy cream that this light bright veggie pasta is a rare treat. Using white wine, lemon, and broth, transfers tons of flavor to the noodles, while not overpowering the taste of the zucchini or squash. The smoked salmon adds the creamy element, meaning you can avoid heavy sauces.

Ingredients:

4 cups zucchini or yellow squash, spiralized

1 package (4 oz), smoked salmon, cut in strips

1/2 cup dry white wine

3 Tbsp. lemon juice, or more to taste

1/4 cup fresh dill, chopped

1 small red onion, minced

3 Tbsp. water

1/2 cup chicken or vegetable broth

8 ounces frozen, peas, thawed and drained

1 lemon, cut in wedges

Directions:

1. Spiralize the zucchini or squash.

2. Blanche noodles, drain and place in a large bowl.

3. In a large skillet, sauté the onion until it is soft and translucent, adding up to 3 Tbsp. water as needed to release.

4. Add the white wine and lemon juice to the skillet, reduce heat, and simmer until it is reduced in volume and beginning to thicken.

5. Add the peas and the broth, stirring gently.

6.   Simmer for 3 more minutes, then add the salmon and dill.

7.   Heat through and stir until the sauce has thickened a little more.

8.   Pour the sauce over the pasta in the serving bowl and toss to blend.

9.   Serve immediately, garnished with lemon wedges.

Note: This dish can be made with canned or leftover poached salmon if you prefer.

Nutritional Info: Calories: 239, Sodium: 273 mg, Dietary Fiber: 8.7, Total Fat: 4.5 g, Total Carbs: 25.8 g, Protein: 25.7 g

---

SPICY SHRIMP WITH VEGETABLE NOODLES AND BABY SPINACH

Servings: 2-3 | Cooking time: 15 minutes | Assembly time: at least 2 hours (for marinade)

Spinach and vegetable noodles provide the perfect background for these tasty little shrimp. Best if grilled on an outdoor grill, it's also possible to use a table-top grill for this recipe. The longer you keep the shrimp in the marinade, the better developed the flavors will be.

Ingredients:

1 large zucchini, spiralized	1 Tsp. Worcestershire sauce
1 large yellow squash, spiralized	3 garlic cloves, crushed
2 pounds large shrimp, peeled and deveined	1 bunch cilantro, roughly chopped, plus more for garnish
1 bunch baby spinach, rinsed well	1/2 Tsp. honey
1/3 cup sriracha	Salt and pepper to taste
1/3 cup vegetable broth	

Directions:

Vegetable Noodles:

1.   Spiralize zucchini and squash. (Thin strands recommended.)

2.   Heat a large pot of lightly salted water to boiling.

3.   Add noodles and blanch for 2-3 minutes until just softened.

4. Drain well.

5. While noodles are still hot, toss rinsed spinach together with them. Heat should be enough to wilt spinach slightly.

Marinade:

1. In a mixing bowl, combine sriracha, broth, Worcestershire sauce, garlic, cilantro, and honey. Add salt and pepper to taste.

2. Reserve 1/4 cup marinade

3. Put in a 1 gallon plastic bag then add shrimp. Mix well.

4. Marinate in the refrigerator for at least 2 hours, longer marinating time will improve flavor.

Assembling the Dish:

1. Heat the barbecue. (If no barbecue available, a table-top grill can be used)

2. Remove the shrimp from the marinade and skewer, filling the skewers within 1/2 inch of each end.

3. Grill each skewer until pink, approximately 3-5 minutes a side.

4. Toss vegetable mixture with reserved marinade until lightly coated.

5. Serve shrimp skewers on a bed of vegetable noodles and spinach.

Nutritional Info: Calories: 554, Sodium: 695 mg, Dietary Fiber: 5.0, Total Fat: 25.1 g, Total Carbs: 24.4 g, Protein: 62.8 g

SPICY VEGETABLE NOODLES WITH KALE AND PEANUT SAUCE

Servings: 1 | Cooking time: 10 minutes | Assembly time: 20 minutes

This recipe adapts well to any taste. Like it a bit spicer? Add more sriracha. Like a bit more creaminess? Increase the peanut butter. Prefer a more fresh taste? More green scallions and kale! Whatever you do to it, the core dish remains the same, and just as delicious.

Ingredients:

1 medium zucchini, spiralized

1 medium yellow squash, spiralized

1/2 Tsp. sesame oil (if desired)

2 Tsp. gluten free soy sauce

1 Tsp. sriracha

1/4 Tsp. fish sauce, plus more to taste

2 Tbsp. peanut butter

1/2 bunch kale, deribbed and sliced into bite-sized pieces

Chopped scallions

For garnish Chili flakes for garnish

Chopped peanuts for garnish

Directions:

Noodles:

1. Spiralize zucchini and squash.

2. Heat a large pot of lightly salted water to boiling. Add vegetables and boil till just soft, about 5 minutes. Remove from heat, and drain, reserving 3 Tbsp. of water.

Sauce:

1. In a frying pan over medium-low heat, mix sesame oil, soy sauce, sriracha, and fish sauce.

2. Stir to combine. Let cook for about 30 seconds. Add peanut butter stir well, and then turn off heat.

3. Assembling the Dish:

4. Heat a large pot of water to boiling. Add kale and blank for 15-30 seconds, until just softened.

5. Drain well and add to the pan of sauce. Add vegetable noodles.

6. Add 1-3 Tbsp. of reserved water, until sauce is desired thickness.

7. Garnish with chopped scallions, peanuts, and chili flakes.

Nutritional Info: Calories: 340, Sodium: 1,914 mg, Dietary Fiber: 7.5 g,

Total Fat: 19.3 g, Total Carbs: 31.5 g, Protein: 17.5 g

SQUASH AND ZUCCHINI PASTA WITH PROSCIUTTO, SNAP PEAS, AND MINT

Servings: 4 | Cooking time: 20 minutes | Assembly time: 15 minutes

This cream-based sauce is both delicious and fresh. The addition of peas and mint keeps it surprisingly light, regardless of the density of the base. The sauce will stay fairly thin, so be aware you might need to cook it down more than you expect.

Ingredients:

½ pound zucchini, spiralized

½ pound yellow squash, spiralized

4 garlic cloves, minced finely

3 Tbsp. olive oil

¼ pound prosciutto, finely diced

4 shallots, minced finely

½ pound fresh snap peas, whole, coarsely chopped

½ cup fresh mint, chopped

Salt and pepper to taste

½ cup cream ¼ cup shredded parmesan cheese

Directions:

Zucchini And Squash:

1. Spiralize zucchini and yellow squash.

2. Bring a large saucepan of lightly salted water to a boil, add zucchini and squash and blanch until just tender, 3-4 minutes.

3. Add peas to water, and boil and addition 1-2 minutes till slightly tender but crunchy.

4. Drain well and set aside.

Sauce:

1. In a heavy sauce pan, cook the prosciutto until just crispy and the fat is beginning to render out.

2. Add the garlic and cook for 2-3 minutes, until just beginning to brown.

3. Add the shallots and cook for 3-4 minutes, until shallots begin to soften and turn translucent.

4. Add several pinches of salt and pepper.

5. Add cream, and bring to a boil, stirring constantly.

Assembling The Dish:

1. Toss vegetables in sauce until well coated.

2. Toss in Parmesan cheese.

3. Dish into bowls, sprinkle with fresh mint, and black pepper.

SQUASH NOODLES WITH TOMATOES AND TURKEY BACON

Servings: 6 | Prep time: 10 minutes | Cooking time: 15 minutes

With bacon, a little bit goes a long way. This recipe is best when tomatoes are in season. Use sungolds for added sweetness or traditional cherry for a more acidic note. Be careful not to allow the arugula to wilt too much, as it will get soggy.

Ingredients:

4 cups yellow squash, spiralized

1 basket cherry tomatoes, halved (or 1 lb. Roma tomatoes, seeded and diced)

1 bunch arugula, trimmed and torn into pieces

1/2 pound turkey bacon

1 large yellow onion, chopped

4 garlic cloves, minced

1 1/2 cups chicken stock

1/2 cup dry white wine

1 Tbsp. Italian seasoning

1 Tsp. crushed red pepper flakes

Directions:

1. Spirlize the squash.

2. In a large skillet, sauté the bacon until crisp. Drain and set aside.

3. Drain the pan well, but do not wipe out.

4. Sauté the onion in the same pan until golden brown, then add the garlic and cook until fragrant.

5. Add the wine and stir, deglazing the pan by scraping up the browned bits of the onion, garlic, and bacon.

6. Add the chicken stock, the tomatoes, crushed red pepper, and Italian seasoning.

7. Cook until the tomatoes are heated through.

8. Add the squash noodles and the cooked bacon. Add the arugula and stir until wilted.

9. Toss with tongs until everything is mixed. Serve immediately.

Nutritional Info: Calories: 394, Sodium: 1,634 mg, Dietary Fiber: 2.9 g,

Total Fat: 24.1 g, Total Carbs: 13.2 g, Protein: 23.9 g

SQUASH SAUTÉ

Servings: 8 | Prep Time: 25-30 minutes

We find this recipe works best with the slightly sweet rich flesh of the summer squash as opposed to heartier winter squashes. The pairing of squash with onions and tomatoes makes it slightly Italian in taste, without being overbearingly like pasta sauce. Still, if you enjoy that, add a little more tomatoes and serve over zucchini noodles and you have a power-packed squash pasta!

Ingredients:

2 lbs. summer squash, spiralized

1 pound ripe Roma tomato, thinly sliced

1 medium yellow onion, thinly sliced

3 Tbsp.s chicken broth

2 Tbsp. large garlic, minced

1/2 Tsp. dried red pepper flakes, crushed

1 Tbsp. Italian seasoning

Parmesan cheese, for garnish

Directions:

1. Spiralize the squash.

2. Heat the broth in a large skillet. Sauté the onion and garlic until the onion is translucent.

3. Add the tomatoes and sauté until the tomatoes have released their juices.

4. Add the squash and sauté for another 1-2 minutes.

5.   Stir in the Italian seasoning and the pepper flakes.

6.   Serve hot.

Nutritional Info: Calories: 49, Sodium: 27 mg, Dietary Fiber: 2.2 g, Total Fat: 1.0 g, Total Carbs: 9.5 g, Protein: 2.1 g

---

Sweet Potato Pasta with Asparagus and Pancetta

Servings: 4 | Prep time: 10 minutes | Cooking time: 7-10 minutes

Pancetta is a fatty rich pork product which combined with asparagus, creates unforgettable flavor. Served over potato pasta, it is fresh, delicious, and just a bit decadent.

Ingredients:

4 cups sweet potato, spiralized

1/4 lb. turkey bacon

1 lb. asparagus, trimmed and cut into 1-inch pieces at an angle

2 medium yellow onions, diced

3 garlic cloves, minced

2 Tbsp. lemon zest (2 medium lemons)

1 Tsp. black pepper

Directions:

1. Spiralize sweet potato into thick strands. Blanche for 5-7 minutes, being careful not to overcook (strands will fall apart if overcooked)

2. Sauté the turkey bacon over medium heat in a large skillet until it is not quite crisp.

3. Drain well, but do not wipe out the pan, then the asparagus and onion.

4. Continue to sauté until the asparagus is tender/crisp (4-5 minutes).

5. Add the garlic, lemon zest, and the pepper. Continue to cook for another 1-2 minutes.

6. Season with pepper.

7. Pour the sauce over the sweet potato pasta and mix.

8. Serve immediately.

Nutritional Info: Calories: 279, Sodium: 225 mg, Dietary Fiber: 9.0 g, Total Fat: 2.0 g, Total Carbs: 53.2 g, Protein: 12.9 g

---

TOMATO-BACON SQUASH PASTA

Servings: 4 | Prep Time: 40 minutes

Bacon is one of the hippest ingredients right now and this pasta uses it to best advantage. If you like your greens a bit crispier, don't cook the pasta after you mix them in, just let the heat of the pasta wilt them.

Ingredients:

2 cups yellow squash, spiralized

1 basket cherry tomatoes, halved

4 strips turkey bacon, chopped into small pieces

1 large red onion, chopped

4 garlic cloves, minced

1/2 cup white wine

1 1/2 cups chicken stock

1/2 cup fresh arugula, chopped

2 Tbsp. Italian seasoning

Directions:

1. Spiralize the squash.

2. In a large skillet, fry the bacon. Remove the bacon and drain off as much fat as possible, but do not rinse out the pan. Add the onion to the pan and cook until it begins to turn golden, then add the garlic and continue to cook.

3. Add the white wine. Deglaze the pan (scraping up the caramelized bits with a wooden spoon and stirring them into the sauce).

4. Add the chicken stock and tomatoes. Cook for several minutes until the tomatoes are heated through then add the Italian seasoning.

5. Crumble the bacon back into the pan and add the noodles, stirring to combine everything. Add the arugula and cook another few minutes until the greens wilt.

6. Serve immediately.

Nutritional Info: Calories: 179, Sodium: 737 mg, Dietary Fiber: 1.5, Total Fat: 10.4 g, Total Carbs: 8.1 g, Protein: 8.8 g

---

Red Wine-Braised Short Ribs with Roasted Turnips

Servings: 3-4 | Prep time: 30 minutes | Cooking time: 2 1/2 hours

This rich wintery recipe is great for cold weather. It may take a little while to cook, but the result is completely worth it and packs a punch. The more fat that renders out of the meat, the meatier your turnips will be. Adjust the amount of oil you add based on the amount of drippings you get.

Ingredients:

4-5 large turnips, spiralized

5 pounds bone-in beef short ribs, cut crosswise into 2 inch pieces

1 Tbsp. olive oil

Kosher salt and freshly ground black pepper

3 medium onions, chopped coarsely

3 medium carrots, peeled, chopped coarsely

2 celery stalks, chopped coarsely

3 Tbsp. almond or rice flour

1 Tbsp. tomato paste

1 750-ml bottle dry red wine (preferably Cabernet Sauvignon)

10 sprigs flat-leaf parsley

8 sprigs thyme

4 sprigs oregano

2 sprigs rosemary

2 fresh or dried bay leaves

1 head of garlic, halved crosswise

4 cups beef stock or broth

Directions:

Roasted Turnips:

1. Spiralize turnips.

2. Preheat oven to 350° F.

3. Toss cut turnips with 1 Tbsp. olive oil and salt & pepper to taste. Spread on baking sheet in a single layer.

4. Place in oven and bake till top just begins to turn golden, 10-15 minutes. Flip with a spatula.

5. Bake other side till turnips are uniformly cooked and softened to the touch (5-10 minutes).

6. Take out of oven and set aside.

Short Ribs:

1. Heat a large heavy-bottomed oven-safe skillet over medium heat.

2. Taking care not to crowd the ribs, cook it in batches over medium heat and brown on all sides. This will take about 10 minutes per batch.

3. Put ribs on a plate and set aside.

4. Drain the pan well, but do not wipe out.

5. Add onions, carrots, and celery.

6. Cook over medium heat until onions are beginning to brown (6-10 minutes).

7. Add flour and mix well, cooking till raw smell goes away, about 5 minutes.

8. Add tomato paste and mix well, cook for 2-3 minutes, until very well mixed.

9. Stir in wine.

10. Add short ribs and any juice that has gathered on the plate.

11. Bring the pot to a boil, then lower heat to medium and simmer for about 25 minutes, until sauce is reduced by half.

12. Add the parsley, thyme, oregano, rosemary, bay leaves, and garlic.

13. Bring to a boil, and then move pot to oven.

14. Cook until ribs are tender, about 2 ½ hours.

15. Take ribs from stock and put on a platter.

16. Strain sauce through a strainer, then remove all solids and discard.

17. Spoon all fat from surface of stock.

18. Put roasted turnips on plates, top with short ribs and stock.

Nutritional Info: Calories: 2,556, Sodium: 1,215 mg, Dietary Fiber: 8.3,

Total Fat: 212.6 g, Total Carbs: 32.8 g, Protein: 87.4 g

TURKEY PHO

Servings: 2 | Cooking time: 45 minutes | Assembly time: 20 minutes

A variation on a traditional Vietnamese dish, this soup features a flavorful clear broth filled with delicious ingredients. Traditional pho uses noodles instead of vegetables, which makes the dish much heavier. The use of squash and zucchini keeps it light and healthy, while still embracing all the tastes of the broth. Err on the side of caution with the honey, as it's much sweeter than sugar. Also, be careful with the fish sauce as it adds a lot of salt!

Ingredients:

2 large zucchinis, spiralized

2 large yellow squashes, spiralized

2 Tbsp. coriander seed

4 whole cloves

4 whole star anise

1 cinnamon stick

1 quart turkey stock

1 bunch green onions (just the green tops), chopped

1/2 Tsp. honey

1-3 inch piece fresh ginger, sliced thinly and crushed

1 Tbsp. gluten free fish sauce (plus more to taste)

1-2 cups kale, deveined and chopped into bite sized pieces

1/2 pound turkey breast or turkey meat, shredded

1-2 Tbsp. cilantro, chopped (for garnish)

1-2 Tbsp. green onions (white bottoms) sliced thinly, for garnish

1/2 lime, cut into wedges

Sriracha sauce

Directions:

Prepare the Zucchini Noodles:

1. Spiralize the zucchini and yellow squash. Set aside.

2. Toast the Spices:

3. Heat a cast-iron skillet or heavy bottomed frying pan over medium heat. Add the coriander, cloves, anise, and cinnamon and toast until fragrant, about 3-4 minutes. Watch carefully to avoid burning.

4. Remove from heat and set aside.

Prepare the Pho:

1. In a large soup pot, mix the toasted spices, stock, fish sauce, ginger, honey, and green onions.

2. Bring to a boil.

3. Reduce heat and simmer 20 minutes on medium heat, skimming froth from surface frequently.

4. After 20 minutes, taste and add honey or fish sauce as desired.

5. Strain the broth and discard solids.

6. Return to heat, and add the kale.

7. Cook for 1-2 minutes until kale is wilted.

8. Add the shredded turkey.

9. Add the zucchini and squash noodles, cook for 1-2 minutes till squash has just softened.

10. Remove from heat, and allow to sit 1-2 more minutes till noodles are in desired texture.

11. Ladle into bowls, add cilantro, onion and sriracha to taste.

12. Serve with lime wedges.

Nutritional Info: Calories: 322, Sodium: 5,203mg, Dietary Fiber: 10.2, Total Fat: 3.3 g, Total Carbs: 40.8 g, Protein: 31.6 g

---

TURKEY PIE WITH SPAGHETTI CRUST

Servings: 4 | Prep Time: 55 minutes

Many recipes like this one call for a lot of extra butter or oil to make the crusts or to sauté onions in. This recipe solves that problem by replacing the butter with chicken stock. Not only is the taste richer, it cuts the excess fat. Just be careful with the salt, as stock will make the recipe a little saltier.

Ingredients:

2 cups zucchini, spiralized

1/4 pound lean ground turkey (can use Italian seasoned if desired)

1 egg, beaten

1/4 cup fresh grated Parmesan cheese

1 cup cottage cheese

4 Tbsp. chicken stock, divided

1 egg, beaten

2 Tbsp. grated Parmesan cheese

2/3 cup low fat, cottage or ricotta cheese

1/2 cup each diced onion &, green pepper

1 cup canned Italian tomato (with liquid), drained & chopped, reserving liquid

1/4 cup tomato sauce

1 Tsp. each sugar & oregano

1/2 Tsp. salt

Dash of each garlic powder & pepper

4 ounces low-fat mozzarella cheese, shredded

Directions:

1.   Spiralize zucchini.

2.   Preheat oven to 350° F.

3. Coat 9" pie pan with non-stick cooking spray. Set aside.

4. In 1 quart bowl combine spaghetti, egg, Parmesan cheese, and 2 Tbsp. stock mixing well.

5. Press spaghetti mixture over bottom and up side of sprayed pan to form a crust. Spread cottage or ricotta cheese over crust.

6. In a skillet, sauté onion and green pepper in 2 Tbsp. stock until soft.

7. Add remaining ingredients except mozzarella cheese. Stir to combine.

8. Reduce heat and simmer about ten minutes.

9. Spread mixture evenly over cottage cheese. Bake 15 to 20 minutes. Sprinkle pie with mozzarella and bake until lightly brown, about 5 minutes longer.

10. Remove from oven and let stand for 5 minutes before slicing.

Nutritional Info: Calories: 425, Sodium: 1,189 mg, Dietary Fiber:, Total Fat: 18.8 g, Total Carbs: 24.4 g, Protein: 38.0 g

---

Turkey Ragu and Potato Pasta Bake

Servings: 4 | Prep Time: 55 minutes

A simple & easy to prepare casserole, this dish is reminiscent of lasagna but without the pasta noodles. The potatoes soak up a bit more liquid than traditional pasta, so the dish will be a little dryer and easier to cut. It freezes very well, just cover tightly and put it in the freezer after layering, remove later and thaw completely, then bake!

Ingredients:

4 large white potatoes, spiralized

1 1/2 pounds ground turkey

1 large yellow onion, chopped coarsely

3 large garlic cloves, minced

1/3 cup dry red wine

29 ounces cans "Italian style" diced tomatoes

1 large carrot, coarsely chopped

2 Tbsp. Italian seasoning

Directions:

1. Preheat oven to 350° F.

2. Spiralize potatoes into thick strands.

3. In a large saucepan add the meat, onion, garlic, and carrot. Sauté until meat is no longer pink, about 8 minutes. Drain very well.

4. Add wine and cook for 3-5 minutes until it evaporates, stirring constantly.

5. Stir in the tomatoes (juice included) and the Italian seasoning.

6. Reduce heat, cover the pan and simmer until the sauce has thickened (about 25 minutes).

7. Spray a glass-baking dish with cooking spray.

8. Layer potatoes in a thin layer over bottom of a baking pan. Spoon ragu in a thin layer over top. Repeat layering until all the ingredients have been used.

9. Bake in oven 30-45 minutes until potatoes are tender.

Nutritional Info: Calories: 650, Sodium: 794 mg, Dietary Fiber: 11.7, Total Fat: 19.1 g, Total Carbs: 70.1 g, Protein: 56.6 g

VEGETABLE MOCK-FRIED "RICE"

Servings: 2 | Prep Time: 10-15 minutes

With just a hint of oil used for flavor and frying the almonds, this dish is a great substitute for more traditional fried rice. Don't hesitate to experiment! Try different veggies you like. We recommend bell peppers and pineapple.

Ingredients:

2 cups cauliflower heads, spiralized

2 whole green onions, chopped

1 cup frozen or fresh snow peas

1/2 cup frozen corn

1 small green pepper, diced

1 small carrot, diced

1 1/2 gluten free soy sauce

2 Tsp. grated ginger

2 -3 garlic cloves, minced

1/4 Tsp. cayenne pepper

1/2 cup raw & unsalted sliced almonds

1 Tbsp. sesame oil

Directions:

1. Spiralize the cauliflower into "rice."

2. Heat a wok or heavy frying pan until very hot. Add oil and stir-fry the sliced almonds for 15 seconds.

3. Add the vegetables and stir-fry for another two minutes.

4. Add the "rice" and stir-fry for three minutes.

5. Add the spices and garlic.

6. Stir-fry for another five minutes, until all ingredients are very hot.

Nutritional Info: Calories: 385, Sodium: 633 mg, Dietary Fiber: 12.2, Total Fat: 21.6 g, Total Carbs: 39.4 g, Protein: 15.3 g

---

Zucchini Pasta Ala Checca

Servings: 2 | Prep Time: 15 minutes

A great make-ahead recipe, this easy sauce is best if you let it sit for a long time. It's easy to mix up and leave in the fridge till you're ready to use it. Best of all, it's fresh, bright, and low-fat! Unlike some sauces that need heavy oils, this pasta relies on the lightness of the tomatoes and basil to taste great without being high in calories.

Ingredients:

4 large zucchini, spiralized

6 large ripe Roma tomatoes, diced

6-8 fresh basil leaves, roughly chopped

4 green onions, diced (white parts only)

2 large garlic cloves, minced

1 Tbsp. grated Parmesan cheese

Freshly ground pepper

Directions:

1. Combine all the ingredients except the zucchini in a glass or ceramic bowl. Cover and allow to stand at room temperature for two hours to blend flavors.

2. Spiralize the zucchini.

3. Warm the strands by quickly dunking them in a pot of boiling water.

4. Drain pasta and top with room-temperature sauce.

5. Toss to distribute the sauce evenly throughout the pasta.

6.   Serve immediately.

Nutritional Info: Calories: 249, Sodium: 182 mg, Dietary Fiber: 15.6, Total Fat: 4.2 g, Total Carbs: 43.2 g, Protein: 18.4 g

---

GREEK LAMB WITH RICED CAULIFLOWER

Servings: 8-10 | Cooking time: 30 minutes | Assembly time: 15 minutes

A rich, tomato dish, the lamb adds its own fats and oils and reduces the necessity of adding additional elements, while retaining the rich, mutton flavor. There are no elements that need to be modified or removed, because all the ingredients are naturally gluten free! In addition, the spices in this dish make it both Mediterranean and delicious, packed with flavor but not calories.

Ingredients:

1 head cauliflower, spiralized

1 pound ground lamb

1 large yellow onion, chopped finely

6 garlic cloves, thinly sliced

2 Tsp. cinnamon

1 Tsp. dried oregano

1 1/2 Tsp. ground cumin

2 Tsp. ground coriander

1/2 Tsp. crushed red pepper flakes

28 ounces can whole peeled tomatoes, drained and mashed

14 ounces can chopped/diced tomatoes

2 cups water

5 ounce (1 bunch) fresh spinach, chopped

2 cups chopped fresh parsley

1/4 cup lemon juice

Salt and pepper to taste

1/4 cup kalamata olives, pitted and finely chopped

1/4 cup crumbled feta cheese

Directions:

Lamb:

1. In a heavy bottomed pan, add ground lamb and sprinkle with 1/2 Tsp. salt and several pinches black pepper.

2. Stir to break apart and cook until nicely browned.

3. Remove from pan and drain well, but do not wipe out pan.

4. Return the pot to the stove, add onions and garlic. Cook until softened and starting to turn color (about 5 minutes).

5. Stir in cinnamon, oregano, cumin, coriander, and red pepper. Cook until toasted and fragrant (1-2 minutes).

6. Stir in mashed tomatoes.

7. Cook tomatoes, spices, onions, and garlic, stirring occasionally for 10 minutes.

8. Add diced tomatoes and 2 cups water.

9. Bring to a boil, then turn down and simmer uncovered for 15 minutes.

10. Add the lamb back to the pot, cover and cook for 20 minutes, stirring occasionally.

11. Stir in spinach, cook for 1-2 minutes until spinach is wilted.

12. While cooking, prepare cauliflower.

Cauliflower:

1. Spiralize the cauliflower into "rice."

2. Heat a large skillet on medium-high with 1 Tbsp. olive oil to coat the pan.

3. Add cauliflower rice and sauté until just turning brown, then remove from heat about 5-8 minutes.

4. Toss cauliflower with lemon juice, and parsley. Add a little water if needed for consistency.

5. ## Assembling the Dish:

6. Spread the cauliflower rice on a large serving dish

7. Top with tomato/lamb mixture

8. Sprinkle with olives and feta to serve.

Nutritional Info: Calories: 296, Sodium: 389 mg, Dietary Fiber: 6.7, Total Fat: 15.3 g, Total Carbs: 23.7 g, Protein: 19.3 g

---

14

DESERTS

"Dessert is probably the most important stage of the meal, since it will be the last thing your guests remember before they pass out all over the table."

William Powell

APPLE CRISP

Servings: 8 | Prep Time: 70 minutes

So many deserts are unfriendly to diets, it is great to find one that's both tasty and healthy. The butter in this recipe is replaced with applesauce, which both cuts calories and increases the apple flavor. After baking, you can broil the crisp for 2-3 minutes to really brown the topping.

Ingredients:

6 large apples, spiralized

1/3 cup almond flour

1/2 cup pecans, chopped

1/3 cup whole oats (not the instant kind)

1 1/2 Tbsp. honey

2 Tbsp. molasses

1 1/2 Tsp. cinnamon

1/2 Tsp. ginger

Juice of one lemon

Directions:

1. Preheat oven to 375° F.

2. Spiralize the apples, thick strands recommended.

3. Combine the apples, 1 Tsp. cinnamon, ginger, honey, and lemon juice. Toss until apple strands are coated.

4. In a second bowl, combine the almond flour, oats, molasses, pecans, and remaining 1/2 Tsp. cinnamon. Use a fork to cut the ingredients together until the texture is crumbly.

5. Put the apple mixture into a 10-inch pie pan and cover with the "crisp" topping.

6. Bake at 350° F for an hour until the filling is piping hot and the topping is crisp and slightly

7. Remove from oven and let stand for 5 minutes before serving.

Nutritional Info: Calories: 248, Sodium: 45 mg, Dietary Fiber: 6.0 g, Total Fat: 12.7 g, Total Carbs: 37.4 g, Protein: 2.9 g

---

APPLE RIBBON PIE WITH NUT CRUST

Servings: 10 |Prep Time: 60 minutes

This apple pie is just as good as grandma made, while staying gluten free. The nut crust is crumbly, crispy, and delicious, and the brown sugar filling caramelizes splendidly. Braeburn applies are preferred over red or golden delicious (they may get too mushy).

Ingredients:

6 medium apples, spiralized

2 cups chopped unsalted nuts (walnuts, peanuts,, almonds, pecans)

3 Tbsp. butter

1 Tbsp. honey

1/2 cup brown sugar

1 Tsp. cinnamon

2 Tbsp. rice starch

1 Tbsp. lemon juice

1/2 cup golden raisins, (optional)

Directions:

Crust:

1. Combine nuts, butter, and honey and press into a 9-inch pie pan.

2. Bake at 350 for 10-12 minutes until crunchy but be careful not to burn the nuts.

3. Set crust aside to cool but leave the oven on.

Filling:

1. Preheat oven to 350° F.

2. Spiralize the apples into thick strands.

3. Combine the brown sugar, rice starch, and the cinnamon and mix with the apple strands and raisins if desired.

4. Pour into the pie shell.

5. Bake at 400 degrees for 45 minutes to an hour. Filling will be bubbly and a little caramelize.

Nutritional Info: Calories: 315, Sodium: 32 mg, Dietary Fiber: 5.5, Total

Fat: 17.8 g, Total Carbs: 38.7 g, Protein: 5.5 g

APPLE/RHUBARB COMPOTE

Servings: 6 | Prep Time: 40 minutes

Rhubarb, also called "pie plant" is an excellent addition to desserts. With a little sugar it's sweet, fresh, and delicious. This recipe has no added fat and all the moisture comes from the fruit or fruit puree! Try different purees to change the flavor balance of the dish, such as peaches or pineapple instead of applesauce.

Ingredients:

6 red delicious apples, spiralized

4 rhubarb stalks, cut into one-inch pieces

1/4 cup honey

1 Tsp. vanilla extract

2 Tbsp. applesauce or pureed pears

2 Tbsp. butter

1/4 Tsp. ginger

1/4 Tsp. cinnamon

1/4 cup brandy (optional)

Directions:

1. Spiralize the apples.

2. Combine the applesauce, honey, vanilla, butter, spices and (if using) the brandy in a large saucepan. Cook over medium heat about 5 minutes.

3. Add the apple strands and rhubarb pieces. Simmer for another 15-25 minutes until the fruit is soft and the sauce has thickened. May be served hot or cold.

Note: If rhubarb isn't in season, you can substitute 2 Bartlett pears peeled, cored and cut into bite-sized pieces. Increase the ginger to 1 teaspoon.

Nutritional Info: Calories: 183, Sodium: 31 mg, Dietary Fiber: 5.2 g, Total Fat: 4.2 g, Total Carbs: 39.1 g, Protein: 0.9 g

---

FRIED APPLES

Servings: 4 | Prep Time: 20 minutes

A quick, easy, and tasty dessert, this works particularly well with very tart apples like granny smith. The use of just a little butter and a little applesauce allows you to sauté the apples till they're tender without adding a lot of extra fat to them. If you want a bit more richness, allow the butter and applesauce brown slightly before adding the apples.

Ingredients:

4 cups (about 4) apples, spiralized

1/3 cup granulated sugar

1 Tbsp. butter

3 Tbsp. applesauce

2 1/2 Tbsp. cinnamon

Directions:

1. Spiralize the apples.

2. Heat butter and applesauce in a large skillet over medium heat.

3. Add the apples.

4. Combine the sugar and cinnamon and sprinkle over the apples.

5. Cook, stirring occasionally, until apples are tender (5-8 minutes).

Note: Some cooks serve these almost mushy, like warm applesauce, but the dish is also yummy when the apples remain intact with little caramelized edges from the sugar.

Nutritional Info: Calories: 228, Sodium: 82 mg, Dietary Fiber: 3.7 g, Total Fat: 3.7 g, Total Carbs: 34.2 g, Protein: 0.6 g

SWEET POTATO PUDDING

Servings: 8 | Prep Time: 75 minutes

A little like a sweet potato pie, this casserole-style dessert is easy to make then forget. It's buttery, sweet, delicious, and very, very simple. It can also be made a day ahead and refrigerated till it's time to bake, just let it come up to room temperature before cooking. Ingredients:1 pound sweet potato, spiralized

Ingredients:

3 eggs, beaten

2 cups milk

1/2 cup raisins, plumped in 1/2 hot, water, and drained

3/4 cup pecan, halves

1/2 cup dark maple syrup

3 Tsp. pumpkin spice, mixes

2 Tbsp. butter, melted

1 Tsp. cinnamon

Directions:

1. Spiralize the sweet potatoes into thick rings.

2. Preheat oven to 325° F.

3. Coat an 8 x 8 baking pan with non-stick cooking spray.

4. Combine all ingredients and pour into prepared pan.

5. Bake for an hour.

Note: This can also be made with squash or pumpkin.

Nutritional Info: Calories: 213, Sodium: 104 mg, Dietary Fiber: 2.3 g, Total Fat: 10.2 g, Total Carbs: 26.3 g, Protein: 5.1 g

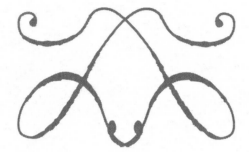

15

NEXT STEPS...

DID YOU ENJOY THIS BOOK?

IF SO, THEN LET ME KNOW BY LEAVING A REVIEW! Reviews are the lifeblood of independent authors, I would appreciate even a few words and rating if that's all you have time for.

IF YOU DID NOT LIKE THIS BOOK, THEN PLEASE TELL ME! Email me at feedback@HHFpress.com and let me know what you didn't like! Perhaps I can change it. In today's world a book doesn't have to be stagnant, it can improve with time and feedback from readers like you. You can impact this book, and I welcome your feedback. Help make this book better for everyone!

ABOUT THE AUTHOR

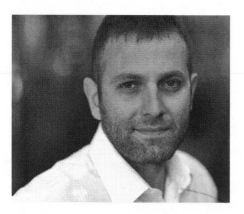

Tom Anderson learned how to cook gluten-free, paleo and weight loss meals out of necessity: a parent developed a severe autoimmune disease which required a significant diet change. Since going gluten-free, he and his family have experienced renewed health, increased energy, and a much happier existence, not to mention new friendships within the gluten-free and paleo communities.

Tom's life changed so radically that he became an evangelist for gluten-free and paleo cuisine. Over the years he has collected, cooked and developed hundreds of recipes which keep his family and friends eager and excited to continue the journey. With the recent introduction of the Vegetable Spiralizer kitchen tool (Paderno Spiralizer, Veggetti Spiral Vegetable Slicer, and a multitude of other Spiralizers), he found a perfect companion to his gluten-free and paleo creations.

Tom lives in San Diego. He cooks when he's not surfing, and takes care of two beautiful daughters and a parent who's health is on the upswing.